5.95

Know Your

Know Your Surgery

Anthony E. Stuart

Consultant General Surgeon and
Surgical Tutor, Oldchurch Hospital,
Romford, Essex

M

© Anthony E. Stuart 1980

First published 1980 by
THE MACMILLAN PRESS LTD
London and Basingstoke
Associated companies in Delhi Dublin
Hong Kong Johannesburg Lagos Melbourne
New York Singapore and Tokyo

Printed in Great Britain by
Unwin Brothers Limited,
The Gresham Press, Old Woking, Surrey

Typeset by
Illustrated Arts, Sutton, Surrey

British Library Cataloguing in Publication Data

Stuart, Anthony E
    Know your surgery,
    1. Surgery — Problems, exercises, etc.
    I. Title
    617'.0076   RD37

    ISBN 0—333—25523—2

FOREWORD

Professor H.D. Ritchie
Surgical Unit, The London Hospital

Although not the first of its kind, Mr Stuart's volume must be the most exhaustive available, at present, to the surgical student. He has put an enormous amount of careful, painstaking work into the preparation of these questions, and yet managed to make it interesting and at times fun to read. Taken in its full depth, it covers more ground than is needed by the undergraduate, and, as the author points out, is adequate to prepare the young surgeon for the final F.R.C.S. examination.

For those whose mind is stimulated by puzzles (self-assessment!), this volume has much to offer. Few, however experienced they may be, will go through many of its pages without discovering some gaps at least in their knowledge.

Mr Stuart is surely to be congratulated in making the results of his careful work available generally to the surgical student.

CONTENTS

INTRODUCTION AND SCORING

This book is designed as a rapid, painless method of both revision and self-assessment in preparing for surgical finals and the F.R.C.S. examination. The material covers the whole range of general surgery and the questions aim to reveal gaps in the student's knowledge and then to help fill these gaps in an entertaining and novel way. Each section is scored and target scores are given to add stimulus and monitor progress.

Although produced for private study, the book may also be effectively used for revision in small groups and will be invaluable for those called upon to teach surgery.

QUIZ QUESTIONS

Forty-five surgical topics are each covered by twenty quiz questions and five multiple choice questions. The former score 1 to 3 points according to their difficulty. Questions with a 3 score are more relevant to postgraduates (P.G.), but some will be in the range of undergraduates (U.G.) and the separate target scores take this into account. A partially correct answer can be marked accordingly, but no half-marks should be scored on the questions with a score of 1.

SCORING THE MCQs

Each correct answer in the five-part questions scores 1 point. For each wrong answer a mark is deducted. An answer left blank does not penalise — zero is scored.

SURGICAL MAZES

These 10 tests are a light-hearted variation on multiple choice questions. Correct answers to true-or-false statements lead to a rapid path through the mazes, whereas two consecutive wrong answers will lead to a back-track, to guarantee you get it right next time!

DIFFERENTIAL DIAGNOSIS COUNTDOWN

Differential diagnosis of important symptoms and signs is important in surgical practice. See how you score on these 330 causes of 60 presenting features.

ACUTE ABDOMEN AND CRYPTIC CASES

Test your surgical knowledge and clinical acumen in diagnosing these 52 simulated case histories. Starting with a presenting complaint and a list of the clinical features available to you, decide what is the most relevant information to reach a correct diagnosis. All of the acute abdomen cases can be successfully diagnosed without turning to the investigations.

To score the case diagnoses start with the presenting complaint and a score of 25 and deduct 1 point for each item of information you require to arrive at the diagnosis (that is 1 point for each page turned to). As soon as you make a diagnosis, write it down with your score and work through the remaining clinical features. Should you need to revise your diagnosis in the light of more information, deduct a further 3 points from your score. Compare your scores with the targets.

TARGET SCORES

QUIZ QUESTIONS

No.	Subject title	U.G.	P.G.	Total	No.	Subject title	U.G.	P.G.	Total
1.	Infection	21	28	41	24.	Vascular — Arterial	18	29	41
2.	Neck	22	30	40	25.	Veins & lymphatics	20	30	43
3.	Thyroid	21	29	41	26.	Fluid	17	26	42
4.	Adrenal glands	19	27	48	27.	Shock	17	26	41
5.	Hernias	21	30	41	28.	Hand surgery	18	28	41
6.	Breast	20	29	39	29.	Orthopaedics	18	27	41
7.	Mouth & pharynx	18	28	42	30.	Fractures	18	27	42
8.	Salivary glands	18	28	43	31.	Head injuries	18	29	45
9.	Oesophagus	21	31	44	32.	Neurosurgery	17	27	39
10.	Stomach	21	30	40	33.	Oncology	18	27	42
11.	Intestine	21	30	40	34.	Thoracic surgery	21	30	49
12.	Appendix	23	32	42	35.	Paediatric surgery	18	28	41
13.	Colon	20	29	39	36.	Plastic surgery	18	28	37
14.	Anorectum	20	30	39	37.	Skin	18	28	41
15.	Liver	19	29	43	38.	Otolaryngology	18	27	40
16.	Biliary system	18	28	40	39.	Gynaecology	17	26	43
17.	Pancreas	21	31	49	40.	Tropical surgery	17	28	43
18.	Spleen	19	28	45	41.	Therapeutics	18	18	39
19.	Kidney & ureter	18	28	38	42.	Biochemistry	21	28	43
20.	Bladder	19	29	44	43.	Anatomy	17	26	41
21.	Prostate	18	29	41	44.	Operative surgery	16	26	38
22.	Penis & urethra	18	28	40					
23.	Testes and scrotum	19	28	37					

MULTIPLE CHOICE QUESTIONS

Each correct answer scores 1 point; for every wrong answer deduct 1 point, any blanks count as 0.

No.	Subject title	U.G.	P.G.	No.	Subject title	U.G.	P.G.
1.	Surgical infection	13	18	24.	Vascular surgery — Arterial	11	17
2.	Neck	10	16				
3.	Thyroid & parathyroid	10	16	25.	Veins & lymphatics	16	21
4.	Adrenal glands	12	17	26.	Fluid	11	17
5.	Hernias	15	19	27.	Shock	14	19
6.	The breast	9	15	28.	Hand surgery	13	19
7.	Mouth & pharynx	14	19	29.	Orthopaedics	13	18
8.	Salivary glands	10	15	30.	Fractures	11	16
9.	Oesophagus	11	16	31.	Head injuries	12	18
10.	Stomach & duodenum	13	18	32.	Neurosurgery	10	15
11.	Intestine	14	19	33.	Oncology	15	20
12.	Appendix	15	20	34.	Thoracic surgery	14	20
13.	Colon	14	19	35.	Paediatric surgery	12	17
14.	Anorectum	10	15	36.	Plastic surgery	14	19
15.	Liver	13	18	37.	The skin	14	19
16.	Biliary system	11	16	38.	Otolaryngology	13	18
17.	Pancreas	11	17	39.	Gynaecology	10	15
18.	Spleen	12	17	40.	Tropical surgery	9	14
19.	Kidney & ureter	13	18	41.	Therapeutics	16	21
20.	Bladder	15	20	42.	Biochemistry	14	19
21.	Prostate	10	16	43.	Anatomy	10	15
22.	Penis & urethra	13	18	44.	Operative surgery	13	19
23.	Testes & scrotum	11	17	45.	Physical signs	7	10

MAXIMUM SCORES FOR ALL PAPERS = 25.

DIFFERENTIAL DIAGNOSIS COUNTDOWN

Countdown	Total	U.G.	P.G.
No. 1	55	45	50
No. 2	55	44	49
No. 3	55	42	47
No. 4	55	43	48
No. 5	55	44	49
No. 6	55	42	47

ACUTE ABDOMEN

Case	U.G.	P.G.	Case	U.G.	P.G.
A	15	18	N	15	17
B	13	16	O	14	16
C	16	19	P	13	15
D	15	18	Q	14	16
E	14	17	R	10	13
F	18	20	S	10	13
G	11	13	T	12	14
H	12	14	U	13	15
I	10	12	V	10	12
J	11	14	W	10	12
K	10	12	X	11	13
L	13	15	Y	12	14
M	14	16	Z	12	14

CRYPTIC CASES

Case	U.G.	P.G.	Case	U.G.	P.G.
A	8	11	N	11	14
B	9	12	O	10	13
C	10	13	P	11	14
D	10	13	Q	12	15
E	10	13	R	12	15
F	11	14	S	13	16
G	9	12	T	10	13
H	8	11	U	9	12
I	7	10	V	10	13
J	10	13	W	13	16
K	11	14	X	9	12
L	12	15	Y	10	13
M	12	15	Z	13	16

SECTION 1

Quiz questions and MCQs

1. How would you treat a boil in a patient who reacts adversely to penicillin? (1)

2. What is the commonest organism to produce acute lymphangitis? (1)

3. What is the commonest organism cultured in gas gangrene? (1)

4. What is the commonest site for a carbuncle? (1)

5. Which condition may result in 'risus sardonicus'? (1)

6. What is the difference between a carbuncle and a furuncle? (1)

7. What are the first symptoms of tetanus? (2)

8. What is the management of a patient with tetanus? (2)

9. How is man infected by hydatid disease? (2)

10. What organism causes a 'malignant pustule'? (2)

11. What are the two commonest sites for actinomycosis? (2)

12. What is erysipelas? (2)

13. What gases are produced in gas gangrene? (2)

14. Where would you expect to find condylomata acuminata? (3)

15. What is the commonest site for hidradenitis suppurativa? (3)

16. What are the features of cervicofacial actinomycosis? (3)

17. What organism classically produces 'empyema necessitatis'? (3)

18. What are the main sites for Ludwig's angina and Vincent's angina? (3)

19. What are the clinical features of amoebiasis? (3)

20. Name two complications of lymphogranuloma venereum. (3)

Target scores U.G. 21, P.G. 28, max. 41

1.   Catch question. You should not treat a boil with antibiotics at all! Lancing and magnesium sulphate paste, if any treatment needed.

2.   Haemolytic streptococcus.

3.   *Clostridium welchii*.

4.   The back of the neck.

5.   Tetanus.

6.   A furuncle is another name for a boil. A carbuncle is a subcutaneous abscess associated with necrosis and multiple sinuses.

7.   Muscle spasms develop in those muscles supplied by same spinal segment as the site of inoculation, then involve the facial muscles producing trismus and 'risus sardonicus', and then the neck and spinal muscles (opisthotonus).

8.   Control spasms by sedation and curarisation, if necessary (with artificial respiration); control of infection by antibiotics and local surgery. Human gamma globulin from fully immunised subjects safer than antitetanus serum.

9.   Contamination from dogs' faeces.

10.   Anthrax.

11.   Cervicofacial and ileocaecal regions.

12.   Diffuse streptococcal infection of the skin and underlying lymphatics. Clear demarcation of the inflamed area and intense local pain.

13.   Carbon dioxide, hydrogen sulphide, ammonia, and hydrogen.

14.   Anus and genitalia.

15.   The axillae.

16.   Bluish indurated swelling over jaw with trismus. Later sinuses discharge thin pus in which 'sulphur granules' may be seen.

17.   Tuberculosis.

18.   Ludwig's angina produces severe oedema of mouth and submandibular region. Vincent's angina produces severe infection of the mouth and pharynx.

19.   Diarrhoea with blood and mucus; intestinal obstruction or perforation; hepatomegaly and, rarely, rupture of abscess into lung.

20.   Complications include inguinal lymphadenopathy progressing to suppuration and sinuses, ulcerative proctitis, rectal stricture and multiple anal fistulae; occasionally elephantiasis.

1.   *Five days after suture of a perforated peptic ulcer a patient develops a temperature of 39°C (103°F). Which of the following would be the likely causes?*:

(a)   Wound infection
(b)   Wound dehiscence
(c)   Pulmonary atelectasis
(d)   Deep vein thrombosis
(e)   Subphrenic abscess

2.   *Tetanus*

(a)   Has an incubation time always less than seven days
(b)   The organisms spread to the central nervous system
(c)   May be mistaken for strychnine poisoning
(d)   Large doses of antitetanus serum are curative
(e)   Severe cases should be paralysed with curare and ventilated via a tracheostomy

3.   *The following statements about a carbuncle are correct*:

(a)   A family history is common
(b)   The back of the neck is a common site
(c)   The condition is commoner in diabetics
(d)   The correct treatment in early cases is systemic antibiotics, and local applications such as kaolin poultice
(e)   It is an area of subcutaneous infective necrosis discharging through multiple sinuses

4.   *Subphrenic abscesses*

(a)   Splinting or paralysis of the diaphragm on screening is usual
(b)   Transpleural drainage should be urgently performed
(c)   Are associated with an ipsilateral pleural effusion
(d)   Are best managed conservatively with prolonged courses of antibiotics (without drainage)
(e)   The commonest type involves the right anterior subphrenic space

5.   *Gas gangrene*

(a)   Is always due to organisms of the *Clostridium* group
(b)   The gas is formed from breakdown of protein
(c)   The organisms may originate in the patient's bowel
(d)   Hyperbaric oxygen is useful in clostridial gas gangrene
(e)   Wide excision of involved tissue is mandatory

Target scores U.G. 13, P.G. 18

1. (a) T   Wound infection is the commonest cause
   (b) F
   (c) F   The fever would have started earlier
   (d) F   Temperature too high for deep vein thrombosis
   (e) T   A subphrenic abscess is not rare after a perforation

2. (a) F   Incubation may be up to several weeks
   (b) F   Only the exotoxin reaches the central nervous system
   (c) T   Both produce tetanic spasms
   (d) F   Antitetanus serum by no means guarantees a cure

   (e) T   This is standard management

3. (a) F   Carbuncles do not run in families — but diabetes might!
   (b) T   Commonest site is the neck
   (c) T

   (d) T   Occasionally surgical drainage is necessary

   (e) T

4. (a) T
   (b) F   Extraserosal drainage should be performed wherever possible
   (c) T   A small pleural effusion above the diaphragm is common
   (d) F   Drainage is required — as well as antibiotics

   (e) F   Although two-thirds of subphrenic abscesses occur on the right,
            the abscess is usually posterior

5. (a) F   Non-clostridial gas-forming anaerobes are not uncommon
   (b) T
   (c) T   Particularly when gas gangrene follows above knee amputation
   (d) T   Hyperbaric oxygen lowers the mortality of clostridial gas gangrene
   (e) T

1.   Name four causes of enlarged lymph nodes in the neck.   (1)

2.   What is the commonest primary source of inflammatory glands of
the neck?   (1)

3.   Give two indications for a tracheostomy.   (1)

4.   Name two complications of tracheostomy.   (1)

5.   Name three causes of a lump in the neck not originating from lymph
nodes or thyroid.   (2)

6.   What is the commonest reticulosis to involve neck glands?   (2)

7.   What are the clinical features of a thyroglossal cyst?   (2)

8.   What is the treatment of a thyroglossal cyst?   (2)

9.   What are the clinical features of a branchial cyst?   (2)

10.   From which cleft does a branchial cyst develop?   (2)

11.   What diagnostic test confirms a branchial cyst?   (2)

12.   Name three causes of a midline swelling of the neck.   (2)

13.   What are the clinical features of a pharyngeal pouch?   (2)

14.   What is a 'sternomastoid tumour'?   (2)

15.   Name two causes of a sinus or fistula in the neck.   (2)

16.   What is a 'collar stud' abscess?   (2)

17.   What are the clinical features of a cystic hygroma?   (3)

18.   What are the clinical features of a laryngocoele?   (3)

19.   What is a carotid body tumour?   (3)

20.   Name two causes of malignant secondary lymph nodes in
the neck with an occult head and neck primary.   (3)

Target scores U.G. 22, P.G. 30, max. 40

1.   There are many causes of enlarged lymph nodes in the neck. The important ones are acute lymphadenitis secondary to pharyngitis or tonsillitis, chronic
lymphadenitis secondary to non-specific or specific infections such as tuberculosis
and glandular fever, primary tumours such as Hodgkin's disease, secondary malignant nodes, for example squamous cell carcinoma from primary head and neck
cancer or secondary to thyroid cancer, carcinoma of the bronchus, breast, etc.

2.   Infection involving pharynx and tonsils.

3.   Examples are (1) airway obstruction, (2) severe laryngeal infection, (3)
laryngectomy for tumour, (4) respiratory insufficiency requiring ventilatioh, for
example severe head and chest trauma, neurological disease, respiratory failure.

4.   Complications include misplacement of the tube, subcutaneous emphysema, pneumothorax, tracheal stenosis, infection.

5.   Swellings include branchial cyst, carot'd aneurysm, affections of the
salivary glands, pharyngeal pouch, lipoma and sebaceous cysts, carotid body tumour.

6.   Hodgkin's disease.

7.   Classically a soft swelling in the midline near the hyoid that moves on
swallowing and possibly on protrusion of the tongue; often brilliantly transilluminable.

8.   Excision of the cyst and thyroglossal tract. If this runs above the hyoid
the centre of the hyoid bone, must be removed.

9.   Classically a branchial cyst presents in young adults as a soft swelling bulging forward from behind the anterior border of the sternomastoid in the upper neck.

10.   The second.

11.   Aspiration with a needle produces a fluid which shimmers with cholesterol
crystals.

12.   Thyroid cyst, adenoma or carcinoma, thyroglossal cyst, dermoid cyst,
sebaceous cyst and lipoma.

13.   Dysphagia localised to the neck, regurgitation of undigested food, foul
breath, gurgling in the throat. Only the large ones produce a swelling, usually on the
left side, presenting from under the anterior border of the sternomastoid; swelling
varies in size according to the contents of the pouch.

14.   Firm swelling in the sternomastoid of neonates associated with torticollis,
probably organising haematoma from birth trauma.

15.   TB, cervical adenitis, branchial fistula, thyroglossal fistula, actinomycosis.

16.   A tuberculous abscess with a small subcutaneous cold abscess communicating through the deep fascia with a larger loculated abscess around tuberculous
lymph nodes.

17.   Multilocular congenital lymph cyst often supraclavicular and brilliantly
transilluminable.

18.   Soft swelling that appears to one side of the larynx on coughing; can be
produced by Valsalva manoeuvre.

19.   Chemodectoma — a tumour of chemoreceptor tissue. |

20.   Characteristic tumours that frequently present with nodes and no obvious
source of the primary are nasopharyngeal carcinoma and papillary carcinoma of the
thyroid.

1.   *Tracheal deviation to the left may be due to:*

(a)   Right tension pneumothorax
(b)   Multinodular goitre
(c)   Collapse of the right middle lobe
(d)   Hashimoto's thyroiditis
(e)   Pericardial tamponade

2.   *A discharging sinus in the anterior triangle of the neck may be due to:*

(a)   Dental abscess
(b)   Osteomyelitis of the jaw
(c)   Branchial fistula
(d)   Actinomycosis
(e)   Thyroglossal fistula

3.   *Tuberculous adenitis:*

(a)   Is always due to *Mycobacterium bovis*
(b)   Frequently requires surgical clearance of infected nodes
(c)   Usually involves posterior triangle glands
(d)   Produces acutely painful lymphadenitis
(e)   Nearly always has associated pulmonary involvement

4.   *Following tracheostomy the patient develops cyanosis. The probable causes might be:*

(a)   Laryngeal spasm
(b)   Glottic oedema
(c)   Mediastinitis
(d)   Tube displacement
(e)   Blockage with secretions

5.   *A man aged 36 presents with painless enlarged lymph glands in the anterior triangle. The cause is likely to be:*

(a)   Tuberculosis
(b)   Syphilis
(c)   Hodgkins's disease
(d)   Hashimoto's disease
(e)   Carcinoma of the lip

Target scores U.G. 10, P.G. 16

1. (a)　T　The mediastinum is pushed to the opposite side
   (b)　T　It may divert the trachea to either side
   (c)　F　Deviation would be to the same side
   (d)　T　The thyroid may be nodular and asymmetrical
   (e)　F　No mediastinal deviation will occur

2. (a)　T
   (b)　T
   (c)　T
   (d)　T
   (e)　T

3. (a)　F　*Mycobacterium* tuberculosis commonly involves neck glands
   (b)　F　Most cases respond to chemotherapy
   (c)　T
   (d)　F　Pain is not a common feature unless secondary infection occurs
   (e)　F　Lymph nodes are frequently involved without active lung infection

4. (a)　F ⎫
   (b)　F ⎬ The obstruction would be above the stoma
   (c)　F　This is a rare cause
   (d)　T ⎫
   (e)　T ⎬ These are common causes of cyanosis

5. (a)　F　Except in an endemic area
   (b)　F
   (c)　T
   (d)　F
   (e)　F

3 THYROID AND PARATHYROID

1.   What is the commonest type of goitre?   (1)

2.   What is an alternative name for infantile hypothyroidism?   (1)

3.   Name three ways of treating thyrotoxicosis.   (1)

4.   Name two antithyroid drugs.   (1)

5.   Name three tests of thyroid function.   (1)

6.   Name three indications for surgery in an enlarged thyroid.   (1)

7.   Name two complications of antithyroid drugs.   (1)

8.   What is the value of a thyroid scan in a solitary nodule?   (2)

9.   What is the replacement dose of thyroxine?   (2)

10.   Name five clinical features of thyrotoxicosis.   (2)

11.   Name three complications specific to thyroid surgery.   (2)

12.   What happens to the serum level of TSH in hypothyroidism?   (2)

13.   Name two clinical tests positive in hypoparathyroidism.   (3)

14.   Name two presentations of hyperparathyroidism.   (3)

15.   What is the usual parathyroid pathology in primary hyperparathyroidism.   (3)

16.   What is the presentation of subacute thyroiditis?   (3)

17.   What is an alternative name for subacute thyroiditis?   (3)

18.   Name three types of thyroid cancer.   (3)

19.   What is the treatment of bony metastases following a follicular
carcinoma of the thyroid?   (3)

20.   What is the characteristic clinical feature of a Riedel's thyroiditis?   (3)

Target scores U.G. 21, P.G. 29, max. 41

1.   Simple colloid goitre, (diffuse or multinodular).

2.   Cretinism.

3.   Antithyroid drugs, subtotal thyroidectomy and radioiodine.

4.   Common drugs are carbimazole, thiouracil, occasionally potassium perchlorate and iodine.

5.   Commonly used tests are protein-bound iodine, radioiodine uptake, serum thyroxine, T.3 resin uptake, serum TSH.

6.   Common indications are pressure symptoms from an enlarged multi-nodular goitre, cosmetic, thyrotoxicosis and suspicion of malignancy.

7.   Skin rashes, gastrointestinal upset, agranulocytosis, hypothyroidism, increase in goitre size.

8.   To distinguish a 'cold' nodule which could be malignant and should be excised. It will also show if a mild thyrotoxic has a toxic adenoma producing a 'hot' nodule with surrounding suppression.

9.   0.1 to 0.3 mg daily.

10.   Features include weight loss, excessive sweating, increased appetite, nervousness, irritability, oligomenorrhoea, diarrhoea, tremor, tachycardia and arrhythmias, exophthalmos.

11.   Hypothyroidism, hypoparathyroidism, damage to recurrent or superior laryngeal nerves.

12.   The serum TSH is very high in hypothyroidism unless it is due to hypo-pituitarism.

13.   Chvostek's sign — tapping the facial nerve, produces twitching of the facial muscles. Trousseau's sign, a blood pressure cuff on the arm maintained above systolic pressure produces paraesthesia and carpal spasm.

14.   Renal calculi and nephrocalcinosis. Bone cysts, particularly in the jaw, bone pain.

15.   Parathyroid adenoma.

16.   Pain and swelling of the thyroid.

17.   de Quervain's thyroiditis.

18.   Papillary, follicular, medullary, anaplastic, lymphoma.

19.   Ablation of remaining thyroid then radioiodine.

20.   Woody hard goitre; adhesion to neck muscles.

1.   *The following features may occur in primary hyperthyroidism:*

(a)   Multinodular colloid goitre
(b)   Diarrhoea
(c)   Anorexia
(d)   High sleeping pulse rate
(e)   Tremor

2.   *Which of the following suggests that a thyroid swelling is malignant:*

(a)   Neck pain
(b)   Hoarseness

(c)   Retrosternal extension
(d)   Palpable lymph glands
(e)   Increased uptake of radioiodine

3.   *Hypoparathyroidism:*

(a)   May result in tetanus
(b)   The commonest cause is thyroid surgery
(c)   Is commonly associated with hyperplasia of all parathyroids
(d)   May result in cataracts
(e)   May require vitamin D therapy

4.   *Which of the following may occur within 48 hours of thyroid surgery:*

(a)   Haemorrhage producing respiratory embarrassment
(b)   Thyroid crisis
(c)   Hoarseness and stridor
(d)   Tetany
(e)   Paraesthesia of the hands

5.   *Hyperparathyroidism:*

(a)   May be due to renal failure

(b)   Can always be diagnosed by an X-ray of the hands

(c)   Is usually due to a parathyroid adenoma
(d)   Commonly presents with renal colic
(e)   Is more common in females

Target scores U.G. 10, P.G. 16

1. (a) F   Hyperthyroidism with a nodular goitre would be secondary
   (b) T   This is a common symptom
   (c) F
   (d) T
   (e) T

2. (a) F   Pain is exceptional in thyroid cancer
   (b) T   Anaplastic carcinomas commonly involve the recurrent laryngeal nerves
   (c) F   Retrosternal extension is as common in benign goitres
   (d) T   Papillary carcinoma commonly involves cervical glands
   (e) F   Most carcinomas are 'cold' on scan

3. (a) F   No, tetany!
   (b) T
   (c) F
   (d) T   This is a well-recognised complication of prolonged hypocalcaemia
   (e) T   Severe cases will not respond to calcium supplements alone

4. (a) T
   (b) T   In an uncontrolled thyrotoxic
   (c) T   From oedema or recurrent laryngeal nerve damage
   (d) T   Due to hypoparathyroidism
   (e) T   This is a premonitory symptom of tetany from hypocalcaemia

5. (a) T   Renal failure leads to phosphate retention and parathyroid hyperplasia
   (b) F   Hand X-rays do not always show subperiosteal decalcification and cyst formation
   (c) T   85 per cent show an adenoma
   (d) T   Renal stone formation is the commonest presentation
   (e) T

1.   Name four clinical features of Cushing's syndrome.   (2)

2.   What is the commonest treatment for Cushing's syndrome?   (2)

3.   What is the commonest cause of a Cushingoid facies?   (2)

4.   What is the sex incidence of Cushing's syndrome?   (2)

5.   What is an alternative name for Conn's syndrome?   (2)

6.   What are the main changes in plasma electrolytes in Conn's syndrome? (2)

7.   How is the diagnosis of phaeochromocytoma confirmed biochemically? (2)

8.   What are the principal hazards of removing a phaeochromocytoma?   (2)

9.   Give two indications for bilateral adrenalectomy.   (2)

10.   Name two tumours of the adrenal cortex.   (2)

11.   Name two tumours of the adrenal medulla.   (2)

12.   Name two surgical approaches to the adrenal.   (2)

13.   Name two techniques to identify the site of an adrenal tumour pre-
operatively.   (3)

14.   What is the macroscopic pathology in Conn's syndrome?   (3)

15.   What is the significance of increased skin pigmentation in Cushing's
syndrome?   (3)

16.   Name one other condition associated with phaeochromocytoma.   (3)

17.   What percentage of phaeochromocytomas are extra-adrenal,
bilateral or malignant?   (3)

18.   Name two clinical features of Conn's syndrome not produced by
hypertension.   (3)

19.   What is the commonest adrenal cause of virilisation?   (3)

20.   What is the commonest cause of Cushing's syndrome in children?   (3)

Target scores U.G. 19, P.G. 27, max. 48

1.   The many features include (1) appearance — obesity, moon-faces, hirsuitism, acne, bruising; (2) complications — hypertension, diabetes, pathological fractures and osteoporosis; (3) general — weakness and muscle atrophy, amenorrhoea.

2.   Total bilateral adrenalectomy.

3.   Treatment with steroids.

4.   Females to males 10 to 1.

5.   Primary hyperaldosteronism.

6.   Hypokalaemia, hypernatraemia.

7.   Urinary vanillylmandelic acid estimation.

8.   There is a serious risk of sudden hypertension or cardiac arrhythmia when the tumour is manipulated, and sudden fall of blood pressure after removal.

9.   Two indications are Cushing's syndrome and metastatic breast carcinoma.

10.   Adenoma; primary and secondary carcinoma.

11.   Phaeochromocytoma, neuroblastoma, ganglioneuroma.

12.   Two principal approaches: (1) the anterior approach through a paramedian, midline or transverse incision; (2) the posterior approach frequently through the bed of the 11th or 12th ribs.

13.   Intravenous urography, presacral gas insufflation and selective arteriography or venography. Selective measurement of adrenal hormones may be helpful.

14.   Most cases are due to an adenoma which is characteristically small, 1—2 cm in diameter, and yellowish on cut section.

15.   Increased skin pigmentation implies a pituitary cause for the Cushing's syndrome, as increased melanocyte-stimulating hormone is being produced.

16.   Phaeochromocytomas can occur in patients with neurofibromatosis. There is also a familial association with medullary carcinoma of the thyroid. Phaeochromocytoma can be part of the multiple endocrine adenomatosis syndrome.

17.   10% in each case.

18.   Muscle weakness, polydipsia, nocturia, carpopedal spasm, and paraesthesia occasionally.

19.   Congenital adrenal hyperplasia.

20.   A malignant adrenal tumour.

1.   *The adrenal cortex*:

(a)   Secretes androgenic corticoids
(b)   Secretes adrenaline and noradrenaline
(c)   Secretes aldosterone
(d)   Secretes glucocorticoids
(e)   Secretes prednisolone

2.   *In Cushing's syndrome*:

(a)   Females are more commonly affected than males
(b)   An adrenal tumour is commonly found
(c)   In over half the cases the pituitary gland shows a malignant tumour
(d)   Hypotension and hypokalaemia are common
(e)   There is increased production of glucocorticoids

3.   *The clinical features of Cushing's syndrome frequently include*:

(a)   Deposition of fat over the face and trunk
(b)   Hypertension
(c)   Diabetes insipidus
(d)   Abdominal striae
(e)   Hirsuitism

4.   *In Conn's syndrome*:

(a)   There is usually hyperkalaemia and hyponatraemia
(b)   The patient is usually hypertensive
(c)   Bilateral hyperplasia of the adrenals is usual
(d)   Selective angiography may be helpful
(e)   A small adrenal tumour is usually found

5.   *Neuroblastoma*:

(a)   Is one of the commonest solid tumours of children
(b)   Frequently presents with haematuria
(c)   May metastasise to the orbit
(d)   May be bilateral
(e)   Arises from sympathetic cells

Target scores U.G. 12, P.G. 17

1. (a)   T
   (b)   F   These are secreted by the medulla
   (c)   T
   (d)   T
   (e)   F   This is a synthetic steroid

2. (a)   T
   (b)   F   Majority of cases are due to adrenocortical hyperplasia
   (c)   F   Cushing's syndrome is rarely due to a benign basophil adenoma
   (d)   F   Hypertension is common
   (e)   T

3. (a)   T
   (b)   T
   (c)   F   Diabetes mellitus!
   (d)   T
   (e)   T

4. (a)   F   Hypokalaemia and hypernatraemia
   (b)   T
   (c)   F   Cortical adenoma secreting aldosterone is found
   (d)   T   This may help localisation
   (e)   T

5. (a)   T
   (b)   F   This is a rare presentation
   (c)   T   This is a well-recognised occasional presentation
   (d)   T   Both adrenals are sometimes affected
   (e)   T   And hence may be extra-adrenal

5 HERNIAS

1.   What is the definition of a hernia?   (1)

2.   What is the commonest hernia in infants?   (1)

3.   What is the commonest external hernia in females?   (1)

4.   Name three factors predisposing to an incisional hernia.   (1)

5.   Which is commoner, right or left inguinal hernia?   (1)

6.   Name two features that distinguish inguinal hernia and hydrocoele.   (1)

7.   Name three differential diagnoses of a femoral hernia.   (1)

8.   What is the anatomical difference between an indirect and a direct
inguinal hernia?   (2)

9.   For what condition is Mayo's operation performed?   (2)

10.   Which adult hernia is most liable to strangulate?   (2)

11.   Which structures are approximated in the usual repair of an   (2)
inguinal hernia?

12.   Which structures are approximated in the repair of a femoral hernia? (2)

13.   What is a sliding external hernia?   (3)

14.   Name two sites of internal hernias (excluding the diaphragm).   (3)

15.   What is the relation of a femoral and an inguinal hernia to the pubic
tubercle?   (3)

16.   Name three surgical approaches to a femoral hernia.   (3)

17.   Name two sites for diaphragmatic hernias (except hiatus).   (3)

18.   What is a Richter's hernia?   (3)

19.   Which abdominal hernia can produce pain in the knee?   (3)

20.   Where do gluteal and sciatic hernias run?   (3)

Target scores U.G. 21, P.G. 30, max. 41

1.   A hernia is a protrusion of a viscus through its coverings into an abnormal situation.

2.   Umbilical.

3.   Inguinal.

4.   Common predisposing factors are obesity, any cause of poor wound healing (for example malignant disease, debility uraemia, vitamin C deficiency, steroids), poor suture techniques or materials, post-operative distension or straining (for example ileus, chest infection, constipation).

5.   The right side in 60 per cent of cases.

6.   A hernia usually demonstrates a cough impulse and reducibility; a hydrocoele transillumination. The examiner can get above a hydrocoele.

7.   Inguinal hernia, inguinal lymphadenopathy, saphena varix, lipoma, and rarely psoas abscess and femoral aneurysm.

8.   The indirect inguinal hernia passes through the deep inguinal ring lateral to the inferior epigastric vessels; the direct medial to the vessels through a deficient wall in the inguinal canal.

9.   Para-umbilical hernias in adults.

10.   The femoral hernia.

11.   The internal oblique and conjoined tendon to the inguinal ligament.

12.   The inguinal ligament to the pectineal reflection of the inguinal ligament or pectineus fascia.

13.   A hernia in which part of the wall of the sac is formed by a viscus that is normally partly extraperitoneal, that is caecum, sigmoid colon and bladder.

14.   Occasional sites for internal herniation are paracaecal fossae, paraduodenal fossae, foramen of Winslow and holes in the greater omentum.

15.   The inguinal hernia originates superior and medial to the pubic tubercle, the femoral inferior and lateral.

16.   Three common approaches to the femoral hernia are: (1) the low approach from below the inguinal ligament; (2) the Lotheissen approach through the inguinal canal; (3) the McEvedy approach through rectal sheath. Bilateral hernias may be repaired through a Pfannenstiel incision.

17.   The foramina of Morgagni (between the sternal and costal origins) and Bochdalek (a defect posterior in the pleuroperitoneal canal). Hernias can occur in central tendon, particularly on the left side.

18.   A hernia in which only part of the bowel wall is strangulated.

19.   An obturator hernia.

20.   Gluteal through the greater sciatic notch, sciatic through the lesser sciatic notch.

5 HERNIAS

1. *An indirect inguinal hernia*:

(a)   Is the commonest external hernia in men
(b)   May be congenital
(c)   Is always associated with muscle weakness
(d)   Very rarely strangulates
(e)   Should usually be treated by a truss

2. *A femoral hernia*:

(a)   Is lateral to the femoral vein
(b)   Is prone to strangulation
(c)   Is more common in females
(d)   Is satisfactorily treated with a truss
(e)   Is usually larger than an inguinal hernia

3. *The following features may be expected in the presence of a strangulated hernia*:

(a)   Abdominal distension
(b)   Fluid thrill in abdomen
(c)   An expansile impulse on coughing
(d)   Local redness over hernia
(e)   Irreducibility

4. *The following predispose to the development of an incisional hernia*:

(a)   Prolonged ileus
(b)   Non-absorbable sutures
(c)   Midline incisions
(d)   Wound infection
(e)   Obesity

5. *Hernias in the umbilical region*:

(a)   Always require operation
(b)   Rarely strangulate in children
(c)   In adults, are commoner in obese females
(d)   Should be treated with an abdominal belt

(e)   Are frequently irreducible in adults

Target scores U.G. 15, P.G. 19

20

1. (a) T   And in women
   (b) T   Due to patent processus vaginalis
   (c) F   Muscle weakness is rare in congenital inguinal hernia
   (d) F   Strangulation is not rare
   (e) F   Surgical treatment is usually advised unless unfit

2. (a) F   Medial
   (b) T   Due to the tightness of the femoral canal
   (c) T   It is uncommon in males
   (d) F   Never!
   (e) F   Femoral hernias are usually small

3. (a) T   Due to intestinal obstruction
   (b) F   The volume of fluid needed to elicit this sign would rarely collect
   (c) F   Strangulation implies incarceration, and hence loss of cough impulse
   (d) T   This is common with strangulation
   (e) T

4. (a) T   Due to tension from distended gut
   (b) F   There are no fewer incisional hernias with absorbable materials
   (c) T   Especially midline lower abdominal incisions
   (d) T   This is a common cause of wound dehiscence
   (e) T   And debility

5. (a) F   Umbilical hernias in babies frequently resolve
   (b) T   Unlike adults
   (c) T
   (d) F   A belt is neither necessary in children, nor advisable in adults, unless
            unfit for surgery
   (e) T   Para-umbilical hernias often have a tight neck and adhesions to the sac

1.   What is the commonest breast lump? (1)

2.   What is the commonest benign tumour of the breast? (1)

3.   Name three common sites of lymphatic spread in breast cancer. (1)

4.   Name three common sites of blood spread in breast cancer. (1)

5.   What is mammography? (1)

6.   What is peau d'orange? (1)

7.   What is cancer en cuirasse? (1)

8.   What is the earliest physical sign that a lump in the breast may be malignant? (2)

9.   Name two conditions producing pain in the breast. (2)

10.   Name three methods of treating bone metastases from breast cancer. (2)

11.   What is Paget's disease of the breast? (2)

12.   What percentage of patients with bony metastases from breast cancer respond to endocrine surgery? (2)

13.   What is the commonest cause of bleeding from the nipple? (2)

14.   What is the commonest cause of a greenish discharge from the nipple? (2)

15.   What would be an indication for giving oestrogen to a patient with breast cancer? (3)

16.   What percentage of clinical stage one breast cancers have positive lymph nodes in the axilla on histology? (3)

17.   What condition can mimic the physical signs of breast cancer? (3)

18.   How does the prognosis of cancer of the male breast compare with female breast cancer? (3)

19.   What might be two causes of severe headaches in a patient with breast cancer? (3)

20.   What is a galactocoele? (3)

Target scores U.G. 20, P.G. 29, max. 39

1.   A cyst as part of fibroadenosis

2.   Fibroadenoma.

3.   Axillary nodes, internal mammary nodes, supraclavicular nodes.

4.   Bones, lung, liver, brain.

5.   A soft tissue X-ray of the breast, to demonstrate early breast cancers.

6.   'Orange-peel' appearance of lymphoedema overlying a carcinoma.

7.   Extensive involvement of chest wall by carcinoma (cuirasse = breast plate, in French).

8.   Tethering to the skin, shown by the demonstration of a dimple on moving the skin over the lump.

9.   Trauma, pregnancy, premenstrual fluid retention, breast abscess, fibro-adenosis; occasionally carcinoma, puberty mastitis and duct ectasia.

10.   Radiotherapy, endocrine ablation, hormone therapy, cytotoxics, methods of pain relief, internal fixation of fractures, etc.

11.   Paget's disease is a red scaly eczematous condition of the nipple associated with an intraduct carcinoma.

12.   30—40 per cent.

13.   A duct papilloma.

14.   Fribroadenosis

15.   A patient with advanced local breast cancer or metastatic cancer who is more than ten years past the menopause.

16.   25—30 per cent.

17.   Traumatic fat necrosis.

8.   The prognosis in males is much worse.

19.   Brain metastases, metastases in the skull or hypercalcaemia, or unrelated causes.

20.   A milk-filled cyst of the breast.

6 THE BREAST

1.   *Common causes of a breast lump are:*

(a)   Cyst
(b)   Carcinoma
(c)   Paget's disease
(d)   Fibroadenoma
(e)   Fibrosarcoma

2.   *Which of the following facts are true about breast lumps:*

(a)   Painful lumps are usually benign
(b)   Nipple inversion always means a carcinoma
(c)   Fat necrosis may produce tethering to skin
(d)   Associated diffuse nodularity suggests fibroadenosis
(e)   Lumps associated with nipple discharge are usually malignant

3.   *Blood-stained discharge from the nipple may be caused by:*

(a)   Duct papilloma
(b)   Galactocoele
(c)   Intraduct carcinoma
(d)   Paget's disease of breast
(e)   Amazia

4.   *Breast carcinoma:*

(a)   Occurs most commonly between the ages of 40 and 50
(b)   Usually occurs in the upper outer quadrant of the breast
(c)   Is the commonest malignant disease of females in the UK
(d)   Usually presents with a painless lump
(e)   At presentation enlarged lymph nodes are found in 75 per cent of patients

5.   *A premenopausal patient with metastatic breast cancer may benefit from:*

(a)   Decadurabolin
(b)   Ethinyloestradiol
(c)   Oophorectomy
(d)   Quadruple chemotherapy
(e)   Subtotal adrenalectomy

Target scores U.G. 9, P.G. 15

1. (a) T
   (b) T
   (c) F   This is a rare lesion and a lump is usually not felt
   (d) T
   (e) F

2. (a) T   Premenstrual breast pain is common with fibroadenosis
   (b) F   It may be congenital or occur in benign disease
   (c) T   Fat necrosis may mimic breast cancer
   (d) T   'Chronic mastitis' is often a diffuse process
   (e) F   Nipple discharge is usually due to a benign lesion

3. (a) T   This is the commonest cause
   (b) F   This is a rare milk-containing cyst
   (c) T   Intraduct carcinoma may mimic a duct papilloma
   (d) T   The weeping eczematous lesion of nipple may bleed
   (e) F   This means absent breast!

4. (a) T
   (b) T   60 per cent are in this site
   (c) T   Causing over 10 000 deaths annually in England and Wales
   (d) T
   (e) F   This figure is too high

5. (a) T   This drug has anabolic and androgenic effects
   (b) F   Being an oestrogen it is likely to be harmful
   (c) T   30–40 per cent of patients respond to ovarian ablation
   (d) T   If hormone treatment fails, chemotherapy may be beneficial
   (e) F   The adrenalectomy would need to be total

1.   Name three types of mouth ulcers.   (1)

2.   What is the primary treatment of most malignancies in the mouth?   (1)

3.   What is the commonest treatment for carcinoma of the tongue?   (1)

4.   What is the commonest treatment for carcinoma of the gum?   (1)

5.   What is the commonest congenital anomaly of the mouth?   (1)

6.   Name two causes of cysts in the jaw.   (2)

7.   What is the surgical significance of the foramen caecum?   (2)

8.   What is the treatment of a mucous retention cyst of the mouth?   (2)

9.   What is the management of malignant glands secondary to oral
carcinoma?   (2)

10.   What is the commonest site for a carcinoma of the tongue?   (2)

11.   Which lip is most commonly involved with carcinoma, and what is the
sex incidence?   (2)

12.   What is the appearance and significance of leukoplakia of the mouth?   (2)

13.   What is the difference between a dentigerous and a dental cyst?   (2)

14.   What is an adamantinoma?   (3)

15.   What is an epulis?   (3)

16.   Name three presentations of carcinoma of the nasopharynx.   (3)

17.   What is a ranula?   (3)

18.   Name three presentations of carcinoma of the maxillary antrum.   (3)

19.   Name a cause for leontiasis ossea.   (3)

20.   What is the commonest type of tumour of the tonsil?   (3)

Target scores U.G. 18, P.G. 28, max. 42

1.   Traumatic, aphthous ulcers, carcinoma, rarely tuberculous, syphilitic, Crohn's, Bechet's.

2.   Local radiotherapy, for example radium implant.

3.   Radiotherapy: radium needles anterior two-thirds, posterior one-third, super-voltage therapy.

4.   Resection of the primary lesion in continuity with mandible and lymph nodes.

5.   Cleft palate and lip.

6.   Developmental cysts, dental and dentigerous cysts, ameloblastomas, bone dysplasias and hyperparathyroidism.

7.   Foramen caecum is the site of origin of the thyroglossal tract; rarely it may be the site for a lingual thyroid.

8.   Excision or marsupalisation.

9.   Monobloc excision — most of these glands are squamous carcinomas and relatively insensitive to radiotherapy, unlike the primary lesion.

10.   Anterior two-thirds, lateral margin.

11.   90 per cent lower lip, 90 per cent males.

12.   White plaques characteristically like cracked white paint. Premalignant.

13.   Dentigerous cyst surrounds an unerupted tooth. A dental cyst forms at the root of a tooth.

14.   This is another name for an ameloblastoma. Multilocular cystic tumour in children or young adults derived from the epithelial cells of the enamel-forming layer, locally destructive, rarely metastasises.

15.   Non-specific term for localised swelling of the gum; three common types — fibrous, giant cell and granulomatous.

16.   This tumour has numerous possible presentations including nasal obstruction and bleeding, deafness, earache, tinnitus, headache, proptosis diplopia and facial paraesthesia. Over one-third of cases present with lymphadenopathy.

17.   Retention cyst of floor of mouth.

18.   Like carcinoma of the nasopharynx this may present in many ways according to the direction of the invasion. Local pain, nasal obstruction, discharge, trismus, toothache, diplopia, facial swelling, lymphadenopathy are examples.

19.   Paget's disease, fibrous dysplasia of bone, rarely syphilis.

20.   Poorly differentiated epidermoid carcinomas.

1.   *The following may predispose to carcinoma of the mouth*:

(a)   Aphthous stomatitis
(b)   Smoking
(c)   Syphilis
(d)   Vitamin E deficiency
(e)   Leukoplakia

2.   *Carcinoma of the lip*:

(a)   Is commonest in middle age
(b)   Occurs more commonly in the lower lip
(c)   The primary requires plastic surgery in most instances
(d)   Is usually painless
(e)   Frequently produces pulmonary metastases

3.   *Cleft lip and palate*:

(a)   A single midline lip cleft is common
(b)   In 15 per cent the cleft lip is bilateral
(c)   In half the cases a cleft of lip and palate co-exist
(d)   The palate is repaired before the lip
(e)   Cleft lip does not interfere with feeding

4.   *Carcinoma of the tongue*:

(a)   Is more common in males
(b)   Commonly presents as an indolent ulcer
(c)   More than half have involved lymph glands at presentation
(d)   Is usually a squamous carcinoma
(e)   Is commonly treated by radiotherapy

5.   *Common swellings in the floor of the mouth are*:

(a)   Sublingual calculi
(b)   Mucous retention cysts
(c)   Submandibular duct calculi
(d)   Adenolymphoma
(e)   Branchial cyst

Target scores U.G. 14, P.G. 19

1. (a)   F
   (b)   T   There is an increased incidence in smokers
   (c)   T   Though a rare cause now
   (d)   F
   (e)   T

2. (a)   F   It is a disease of the elderly
   (b)   T   90 per cent occur on the lower lip
   (c)   F   Radiotherapy is excellent primary treatment in many cases
   (d)   T
   (e)   F   Most metastases occur via lymphatics

3. (a)   F   This is excessively rare
   (b)   T
   (c)   T
   (d)   F   Palatal repair is often delayed until the child is one year old
   (e)   T   Feeding difficulties are rare with cleft lip — unlike cleft palate

4. (a)   T
   (b)   T   Although occasionally the growth may be heaped-up or papilliferous
   (c)   T   These glands require block dissection
   (d)   T   Other tumours are rare
   (e)   T

5. (a)   F
   (b)   T   A large cyst may be called a 'ranula'
   (c)   T   This gland is not infrequently involved by calculi
   (d)   F   This is a tumour of the parotid in older males
   (e)   F   This does not present in the floor of the mouth

8 SALIVARY GLANDS

1. Which gland is most commonly involved with a salivary tumour? (1)
2. What is the commonest type of salivary tumour? (1)
3. Which gland is most commonly involved with a calculus? (1)
4. What is the usual cause of a parotid abscess? (1)
5. What are the symptoms of a submandibular calculus? (1)

6. What is the management of a submandibular calculus? (2)

7. What feature makes a parotid tumour likely to be malignant? (2)
8. Name two malignant varieties of parotid tumour. (2)

9. Name two local complications of operation for parotid tumours. (2)
10. What is the commonest site for metastases from carcinoma of the parotid? (2)
11. What is the operation of choice for a mixed parotid tumour? (2)
12. What are the symptoms of sialectasis? (2)

13. Name three organs that may be involved by mumps other than the salivary glands. (3)
14. What is the commonest cause of Mikulicz's syndrome? (3)
15. What is Frey's syndrome? (3)
16. What is the commonest site of a tumour of the minor salivary glands? (3)
17. What is Sjögren's syndrome? (3)

18. What is an alternative name for Warthin's tumour? (3)
19. What are the clinical features of a Warthin's tumour? (3)

20. Name three different diagnoses of generalised parotid swelling. (3)

Target scores U.G. 18, P.G. 28, max. 43

1.   The parotid.

2.   The mixed parotid tumour (pleomorphic adenoma).

3.   Submandibular gland.

4.   Poor oral hygiene and dehydration.

5.   Intermittent swelling and discomfort in the submandibular gland related to meals.

6.   If the stone is in the duct it should be removed through the mouth. If it is in the gland, the gland itself should be removed.

7.   Involvement of the facial nerve.

8.   Muco-epidermoid carcinoma, squamous cell carcinoma, adenocarcinoma and adenoid cystic carcinoma (cylindroma).

9.   Bleeding, infection, facial nerve damage, parotid fistula.

10.   Cervical lymph nodes.

11.   Conservative parotidectomy (preserving the facial nerve).

12.   Recurrent swelling and discomfort in the salivary glands, usually involving more than one gland (unlike submandibular calculus).

13.   Breast, thyroid, testes, ovaries, pancreas, central nervous system.

14.   Autoimmune disease.

15.   Gustatory sweating in the distribution of the auriculotemporal nerve.

16.   The hard palate.

17.   Enlargement of the salivary and lachrymal glands associated with conjunctivokeratitis and often arthritis in middle-aged females.

18.   Adenolymphoma.

19.   Soft, cystic, slowly enlarging, benign tumour of middle-aged to elderly men. Ten per cent are bilateral.

20.   Sarcoidosis (the commonest), reticuloses, tuberculosis, Sjögren's syndrome, mumps, chronic recurrent parotitis.

8 SALIVARY GLANDS

1.   *A mixed parotid tumour (pleomorphic adenoma)*:

(a)   May turn malignant
(b)   Is slowly growing
(c)   Is usually confined to the deep lobe of the parotid
(d)   Does not occur in the submandibular or sublingual glands
(e)   Commonly produces a facial palsy

2.   *In treatment of a mixed parotid tumour*:

(a)   The whole parotid must be removed
(b)   Enucleation is satisfactory
(c)   Radiotherapy may be used for recurrence
(d)   Suprafacial conservative parotidectomy is the usual operation
(e)   Facial nerve damage occurs in 50 per cent of the cases treated surgically

3.   *Submandibular calculi*:

(a)   May be caused by hyperparathyroidism
(b)   Are frequently formed during an attack of mumps
(c)   Commonly give rise to gland swelling on eating
(d)   Are usually removed by an incision under the chin
(e)   May require removal of the submandibular gland

4.   *Recurrent attacks of parotid swelling may be due to*:

(a)   Mumps
(b)   Sialectasis
(c)   Parotid duct calculi
(d)   Adenolymphoma
(e)   Felty's syndrome

5.   *Carcinoma of the parotid*:

(a)   May be adenocarcinoma or squamous carcinoma
(b)   Has a good prognosis
(c)   Usually requires sacrifice of the facial nerve
(d)   Blood-borne metastases do not occur
(e)   Radiotherapy is the treatment of choice

Target scores U.G. 10, P.G. 15

1. (a) T   Although rare, this is a well-recognised complication
   (b) T   The history may be over years
   (c) F   Superficial lobe is more common
   (d) F   Although less common, both glands may contain this tumour
   (e) F   This is a sign of malignant change

2. (a) F   Superficial parotidectomy is usually adequate
   (b) F   A high recurrence rate will follow
   (c) T
   (d) T   Removal of the superficial lobe covering the facial nerve
   (e) F   Not unless the surgeon has a tremor!

3. (a) F   This is not a recognised complication
   (b) F   There is no evidence that mumps predisposes to stones
   (c) T   This is the common presentation
   (d) F   Duct calculi should be removed through the mouth
   (e) T   Stones in this gland are best treated by gland excision or a fistula may
            follow

4. (a) F   Repeated mumps attacks are very rare
   (b) T   This is the commonest cause
   (c) T   Although less common than submandibular calculi
   (d) F   This is a benign tumour
   (e) F   This syndrome is rheumatoid arthritis with splenic enlargement

5. (a) T   Although the former is commoner
   (b) F   Early invasion and lymphatic spread is common
   (c) T   Radical surgery offers the best chance of cure
   (d) F   Late spread to lungs and bone does occur
   (e) F   The tumour is relatively radioresistant

9 OESOPHAGUS

1.   Name three causes of dysphagia.   (1)

2.   What is the commonest cause of oesophageal perforation?   (1)
3.   Name two causes of dysphagia associated with pain.   (1)

4.   What is the sex incidence of carcinoma of the oesophagus?   (1)

5.   What is the treatment of achalasia of the cardia?   (2)

6.   What is the pathophysiology of achalasia?   (2)

7.   What are the indications for surgery in hiatus hernia?   (2)

8.   Name a method of stopping bleeding from oesophageal varices.   (2)

9.   Name two clinical features of oesophageal perforation.   (2)

10.   What is an alternative name for Heller's operation?   (2)
11.   What is a common complication of achalasia?   (2)
12.   Name two types of oesophageal diverticulum.   (2)
13.   What is the main value of the oesophageal perfusion test?   (3)
14.   Name two pre-malignant conditions of the oesophagus.   (3)
15.   What is the Mallory—Weiss syndrome?   (3)

16.   What condition can mimic the X-ray changes of achalasia?   (3)
17.   In what condition do you see a 'corkscrew oesophagus' on X-ray?   (3)
18.   What is the commonest benign tumour of the oesophagus?   (3)
19.   What is Chaga's disease?   (3)

20.   What is Boerhaave's syndrome?   (3)

Target scores U.G. 21, P.G. 31, max. 44

1.　　There are numerous causes of dysphagia; among the commoner are tonsillitis, pharyngitis, diffuse oesophageal spasm, reflux oesophagitis, achalasia, carcinoma of the oesophagus, carcinoma of the bronchus, retrosternal goitre, mediastinal nodes, aneurysm, pharyngeal pouch, Plummer—Vinson syndrome, scleroderma and neurological causes.

2.　　Iatrogenic causes from oesophagoscopy and bouginage.

3.　　Tonsillitis, pharyngitis, reflux oesophagitis, diffuse oesophageal spasm, foreign bodies, caustic strictures.

4.　　Strong male preponderance except for upper third which is commoner in females and frequently secondary to Paterson—Kelly syndrome, (Plummer—Vinson syndrome).

5.　　Hydrostatic dilatation in early cases, cardiomyotomy (Heller's operation) in more advanced cases.

6.　　Degeneration or abnormality of autonomic nerve ganglia in Auerbach's plexus.

7.　　(1) Failed medical treatment (2) complications of the oesophagitis (that is bleeding, stricture) and (3) all paraoesophageal hernias.

8.　　Intravenous Pitressin, Sengstaken tube, injection or ligation of varices, selective catheterisation and embolisation of regional vessels, portosystemic shunt.

9.　　Chest pain, especially on inspiration and swallowing, surgical emphysema in the neck.

10.　　Cardiomyotomy.

11.　　Aspiration pneumonia, rarely malignant change.

12.　　Pulsion and traction, rarely congenital.

13.　　To distinguish the pain of reflux oesophagitis from cardiac pain.

14.　　Post-cricoid web (Plummer—Vinson syndrome) leukoplakia, achalasia.

15.　　Mucosal tear in the lower part of the oesophagus or upper stomach, secondary to vomiting, producing haematemesis.

16.　　Scleroderma.

17.　　Diffuse oesophageal spasm.

18.　　Leiomyoma.

19.　　Trypanosome infection found in Brazil that produces degeneration of ganglia in the colon and oesophagus, and therefore a clinical picture of achalasia.

20.　　Similar to Mallory—Weiss syndrome except the vomiting produces a complete tear of the lower part of the oesophagus and the clinical picture of an oesophageal perforation.

9 OESOPHAGUS

1.   *Oesophageal atresia*:

(a)   Is a very rare developmental abnormality
(b)   Is usually associated with a tracheo-oesophageal fistula
(c)   Usually presents with failure to thrive
(d)   May present with cyanosis
(e)   Absence of intestinal gas in an abdominal X-ray is diagnostic

2.   *Hiatus hernia*:

(a)   Most hiatus hernias are of the rolling type
(b)   May present with anaemia
(c)   May occur in infancy
(d)   Usually requires operative treatment
(e)   Is always associated with reflux oesophagitis

3.   *Carcinoma of the oesophagus*:

(a)   Is commoner in men
(b)   Usually presents with progressive dysphagia
(c)   Is the commonest cause of haematemesis over 60
(d)   Is best diagnosed by oesophageal manometry
(e)   Is frequently inoperable

4.   *Sideropaenic dysphagia*:

(a)   Usually occurs in middle-aged women
(b)   Parietal cell antibodies are usually strongly positive
(c)   Koilonychia and atrophic oral epithelium are associated
(d)   A web is commonly found in the mid-oesophagus
(e)   Most patients require pharyngolaryngectomy

5.   *Stricture of the oesophagus*:

(a)   The commonest cause is reflux oesophagitis
(b)   Frequently requires colonic replacement
(c)   May follow propanolol therapy
(d)   Usually responds to dilatation treatment
(e)   May be secondary to lye ingestion

Target scores U.G. 11, P.G. 16

1. (a)   F   It is a relatively common congenital abnormality
   (b)   T   Over 90 per cent
   (c)   F   Regurgitation and cyanosis are commonest
   (d)   T
   (e)   F   Intestinal gas is usual as commonly the tracheo-oesophageal fistula communicates with the lower oesophagus

2. (a)   F   Over 85 per cent are sliding
   (b)   T   From oesophagitis or ulceration
   (c)   T   Associated with a lax hiatus
   (d)   F   Most cases are treated medically
   (e)   F   This is uncommon with para-oesophageal hernias

3. (a)   T   Except for the less-common post-cricoid carcinomas
   (b)   T
   (c)   F   This is acute or chronic peptic ulceration
   (d)   F   Barium swallow and oesophagoscopy
   (e)   T   Over half are advanced at presentation

4. (a)   T   Usually secondary to menorrhagia
   (b)   F   There is no relation to pernicious anaemia
   (c)   T   In severe anaemia koilonychia, glossitis and angular cheilosis
   (d)   F   Post-cricoid
   (e)   F   Treatment of the anaemia is usually adequate

5. (a)   T
   (b)   F   Most cases respond to dilatation
   (c)   F   This is not a known complication of propanolol
   (d)   T
   (e)   T   Lye is a caustic substance and, if swallowed, leads to severe stricture formation

1.   What is the commonest site of a benign gastric ulcer?   (1)

2.   Name three complications of peptic ulceration.   (1)

3.   What is the commonest site of a carcinoma of the stomach?   (1)

4.   What is a Billroth I gastrectomy?   (1)

5.   Which has the higher recurrent ulcer rate, subtotal gastrectomy or
vagotomy, in the treatment of duodenal ulceration?   (1)

6.   Name three causes of haematemesis other than chronic peptic
ulceration.   (1)

7.   Name two drugs believed to produce gastric erosions.   (1)

8.   What is the commonest site of a perforated peptic ulcer?   (1)

9.   What is a linitis plastica?   (2)

10.   What is Rammstedt's operation?   (2)

11.   How may one differentiate clinically between pyloric stenosis and
duodenal atresia in infants?   (2)

12.   What is the usual cause of an hour-glass stomach?   (2)

13.   Name three medical measures proven to heal benign gastric ulcers.   (3)

14.   Name two tests of gastric acid secretion.   (3)

15.   Name three types of vagotomy.   (3)

16.   What is the usual cause for a gastrojejunocolic fistula?   (3)

17.   Name a test for incomplete vagotomy.   (3)

18.   What percentage of patients with a perforated duodenal ulcer
have air under the diaphragm?   (3)

19.   What is 'dumping syndrome'?   (3)

20.   What are Curling's and Cushing's ulcers?   (3)

Target scores U.G. 21, P.G. 30, max. 40

1.   Lesser curvature.

2.   Haemorrhage, perforation, pyloric stenosis, penetration of the pancreas, malignant change.

3.   Antrum.

4.   Partial gastrectomy and end-to-end gastroduodenal anastomosis are usually performed for a gastric ulcer.

5.   Vagotomy (usually due to incomplete vagotomy).

6.   Acute gastric erosions, varices, Mallory–Weiss syndrome, gastric tumours, hiatus hernia, bleeding disorders, nasopharyngeal bleeding.

7.   Aspirin, phenyl butazone, indomethocin, steroids.

8.   Anterior duodenum.

9.   'Leather bottle stomach' due to infiltrating submucosal carcinoma.

10.   Pyloromyotomy for hypertrophic congenital pyloric stenosis.

11.   Duodenal atresia produces vomiting from birth, whereas in hypertrophic pyloric stenosis the vomiting characteristically starts a few days to a few weeks after birth. In the former the vomitus contains bile. In the latter, a palpable mass is present in most cases.

12.   Fibrosis from a benign gastric ulcer.

13.   Bed rest, stopping smoking, carbonoxolone, H_2 antagonists.

14.   Histamine test, pentagastrin test, insulin test.

15.   Truncal, selective, highly selective (proximal gastric vagotomy or parietal cell vagotomy).

16.   Recurrent peptic ulceration after previous gastrectomy and gastrojejunostomy. Rarely, a carcinoma of the colon or stomach.

17.   Hollander insulin test, or Burge stimulation test (at time of vagotomy).

18.   80%.

19.   A symptom complex in which the patient develops a feeling of epigastric fullness, sweating, discomfort and faintness after meals. Late dumping may be associated with feelings of epigastric emptiness and hunger.

20.   Both are gastroduodenal stress ulcers, the first due to burns, the second due to raised intracranial pressure.

1.   *In the management of a patient with haematemesis*:

(a)   Age and size of initial bleed give a good guide to prognosis
(b)   Old patients should be treated conservatively for as long as possible
(c)   Early gastroscopy is dangerous and ineffective
(d)   Gastric cooling has doubled survival figures
(e)   Patients should be undertransfused to prevent further bleeding

2.   *The common causes of upper gastrointestinal bleeding include*:

(a)   Scurvy
(b)   Haemophilia
(c)   Aspirin
(d)   Paracetamol
(e)   Ascorbic acid

3.   *A patient with pyloric stenosis may present with*:

(a)   Metabolic acidosis
(b)   Bilious vomiting
(c)   Succussion splash
(d)   Visible peristalsis
(e)   Bluish discoloration in the flanks

4.   *Late complications of partial gastrectomy include*:

(a)   Osteomalacia
(b)   Iron deficiency anaemia
(c)   Steatorrhoea
(d)   Gluten enteropathy
(e)   Carcinoid syndrome

5.   *In the Zollinger–Ellison syndrome*:

(a)   An alpha cell tumour of the pancreas is always found
(b)   Highly selective vagotomy is the treatment of choice
(c)   Diarrhoea may be the presenting feature

(d)   Total gastrectomy may be necessary

(e)   Serum gastrin levels are usually high

Target scores U.G. 13, P.G. 18

1. (a)   T   Mortality is proportional to age and volume of blood loss
   (b)   F   Old age is an indication for early surgery
   (c)   F   Early gastroscopy should be routine
   (d)   F   There is no dramatic improvement with gastric cooling
   (e)   F   The doctrine of keeping the patient slightly shocked is appalling!

2. (a)   F   It is rare
   (b)   F   This, too, is rare
   (c)   T   Aspirin is the commonest cause of drug-induced gastric erosions
   (d)   F   Paracetamol does not lead to gastric irritation
   (e)   F   No

3. (a)   F   Alkalosis would follow prolonged vomiting
   (b)   F   The vomit would be bile-free in pyloric stenosis
   (c)   T   This is characteristic
   (d)   T   In a baby or thin adult visible peristalsis may be seen
   (e)   F

4. (a)   T   Due to prolonged calcium malabsorption
   (b)   T   Slight anaemia is common after gastrectomy
   (c)   T   Increased faecal fats from malabsorption may occur
   (d)   F } Neither of these conditions is associated with gastrectomy
   (e)   F }

5. (a)   F   The syndrome can be due to G-cell hyperplasia in the gastric antrum
   (b)   F   This is an inadequate operation for Zollinger—Ellison syndrome
   (c)   T   The cause is complex but related to the volume of acid entering the small gut
   (d)   T   If the tumour cannot be removed and the ulceration cannot be controlled by Cimetidine, total gastrectomy may be necessary
   (e)   T   Levels are usually diagnostic

1.   What is an intussusception?   (1)

2.   What is the commonest age for an intussusception?   (1)

3.   What is the commonest site for Crohn's disease?   (1)

4.   Name two causes of spontaneous intestinal fistula formation.   (1)

5.   What is the commonest condition requiring an ileostomy?   (1)

6.   What are the two commonest causes of small-bowel obstruction in
adults?   (2)

7.   Name two causes of intestinal obstruction from a blocked lumen.   (2)

8.   Name three causes of intestinal obstruction in neonates.   (2)

9.   Name four symptoms of intestinal obstruction.   (2)

10.   What is absolute constipation?   (2)

11.   What are the features that make one suspect that an intestinal
obstruction is associated with strangulation?   (2)

12.   What condition is classically associated with 'redcurrant jelly' stools?   (2)

13.   Name three complications of a Meckel's diverticulum.   (2)

14.   What is the connection between 5-hydroxyindoleacetic acid (5-HIAA)
and the gut?   (2)

15.   What features on plain abdominal X-ray distinguish a jejunal obstruction
from a lower small-bowel obstruction?   (2)

16.   What is the commonest site for a carcinoid tumour?   (3)

17.   What is the 'string sign' of Kantor?   (3)

18.   What is the usual cause of an intussusception in adults?   (3)

19.   What is the Peutz-Jeghers syndrome?   (3)

20.   Name three primary small-bowel tumours.   (3)

Target scores U.G. 21, P.G. 30, max. 40

1.   The invagination of the bowel within itself. It most commonly occurs in the ileocaecal region.

2.   The commonest age group is 6—12 months of age.

3.   Terminal ileum.

4.   Crohn's disease, diverticular disease, carcinoma of the colon.

5.   Ulcerative colitis, panproctocolectomy.

6.   Adhesions from previous surgery or inflammation, hernias.

7.   Obstruction from inspissated faeces, foreign body, food bolus or gallstone ileus.

8.   Atresia, stenosis, malrotation volvulus neonatorum, anorectal agenesis, Hirschsprung's disease, internal and external hernias.

9.   Colic, distension, nausea and vomiting, constipation, absence of flatus.

10.   Absolute constipation is the term used when the patient is not only constipated but failing to pass flatus.

11.   Tachycardia, fever, tenderness — particularly rebound tenderness, guarding and absent bowel sounds.

12.   Intussusception.

13.   Acute inflammation, ulceration with possible bleeding or perforation. The Meckel's diverticulum may be the cause of an intussusception or volvulus.

14.   Carcinoid syndrome: 5-HIAA is a breakdown product of 5-hydroxytryptamine.

15.   In a jejunal obstruction, lines appear to cross the full width of the bowel lumen. These are the valvulae conniventes. Number of dilated loops.

16.   The appendix.

17.   The gross luminal narrowing seen on barium meal and follow-through in a case of Crohn's disease of the terminal ileum.

18.   A tumour, usually malignant.

19.   An inherited condition in which intestinal polyposis is associated with pigmentation in or around the mouth. The polyps are hamartomas and rarely turn malignant.

20.   Benign examples are leiomyoma, submucous lipoma, adenoma, haemangioma; malignant ones are lymphosarcoma, carcinoid tumour and carcinoma.

1.   *The following are well-recognised complications of Crohn's disease:*

(a)   Erythema multiforme
(b)   Polyarthropathy
(c)   Anal fistula
(d)   Iritis
(e)   Ascending cholangitis

2.   *The following features may occur in carcinoid syndrome:*

(a)   Raynaud's phenomena
(b)   Attacks of flushing
(c)   Diarrhoea
(d)   Bronchospasm
(e)   Pulmonary stenosis

3.   *A patient with high jejunal obstruction will typically demonstrate:*

(a)   Profuse vomiting
(b)   Numerous dilated loops on abdominal X-ray
(c)   Marked abdominal distension
(d)   Hyponatraemia
(e)   Increased bowel sounds

4.   *A man of 46 presents with intestinal obstruction. Which of the following are likely to be the cause:*

(a)   Mesentric infarction
(b)   Gall-stone ileus
(c)   Hernia
(d)   Mesenteric cyst
(e)   Adhesions from previous surgery

5.   *Malabsorption may be due to the following:*

(a)   Chronic pancreatitis
(b)   Obstructive jaundice
(c)   Coeliac disease
(d)   Blind-loop syndrome
(e)   Mallory-Weiss syndrome

Target scores U.G. 14, P.G. 19

1. (a) F   Erythema nodosum can occur
   (b) T
   (c) T   Anal complications occur in 30 per cent of Crohn's patients
   (d) T
   (e) F   Though rarely, sclerosing cholangitis may occur

2. (a) F
   (b) T ⎫
   (c) T ⎬ These are common features
   (d) T ⎫
   (e) T ⎬ Though less common, both may occur in carcinoid syndrome

3. (a) T
   (b) F   With a high jejunal obstruction very few loops will be dilated
   (c) F   Distension is not a feature of high intestinal obstruction
   (d) T   Electrolyte disturbance is often marked
   (e) T   Bowel sounds are usually increased and obstructive unless strangulation
            has occurred or the obstruction is at the duodenojejunal flexure

4. (a) F   This would be rare at this age
   (b) F   This rare cause usually occurs in women
   (c) T   The second commonest cause of small-bowel obstruction
   (d) F
   (e) T   This is the commonest cause of intestinal obstruction

5. (a) T   Owing to reduced exocrine secretion of pancreatic enzymes
   (b) T   From a deficiency of bile salts for fat emulsification
   (c) T   Due to gluten-sensitive enteropathy
   (d) T   From bacterial overgrowth in the blind loop
   (e) F   This condition is bleeding causes by vomiting producing a mucosal tear

1.   What is the typical pattern of pain in appendicitis?   (1)

2.   What type of incision is the commonest approach to the appendix?   (1)

3.   Name two complications of appendicectomy.   (1)

4.   What is an indication for conservative management in appendicitis?   (1)

5.   What is the mortality arising from appendicitis — 1 in 20, 200, 2000, or 20 000?   (2)

6.   What is the commonest position for the appendix?   (2)

7.   When may diarrhoea be a feature of appendicitis?   (2)

8.   What sort of patients are most at risk from appendicitis?   (2)

9.   What is the best guide to the base of the appendix at operation?   (2)

10.   Give three differential diagnoses of an appendix mass.   (2)

11.   Name four important differential diagnoses of appendicitis.   (2)

12.   Name two problems of appendicitis occurring in pregnancy.   (2)

13.   What would be an indication for a paramedian incision in suspected appendicitis?   (2)

14.   Name three complications of appendicitis.   (2)

15.   How does the appendix differ histologically in childhood and old age? (3)

16.   What percentage of individuals in Western society come to appendicectomy?   (3)

17.   What percentage of cases of appendicitis are due to obstruction of the proximal lumen?   (3)

18.   What is the commonest tumour of the appendix?   (3)

19.   How do you treat carcinoma of the appendix?   (3)

20.   What is pseudomyxoma peritonei?   (3)

Target scores U.G. 23, P.G. 32, max. 42

1.   Central abdominal colic, moving to the right iliac fossa and becoming continuous pain.

2.   The grid-iron incision.

3.   Important ones are (1) local — haemorrhage, infection (wound, pelvic, sub-phrenic, rarely liver abscess), rarely intestinal obstruction, fistula formation; (2) general — chest infection, septicaemia, thromboembolism.

4.   Cases presenting late with a palpable mass but no signs of generalised peritonitis.

5.   1 in 200, mostly elderly.

6.   Retrocaecal.

7.   When the appendix is pelvic or retro-ileal. Diarrhoea is more common in children with appendicitis.

8.   The very young and the very old. In both groups the diagnosis is often made late, perforation is more common and resistance to infection impaired.

9.   The taeniae coli converge on the base of the appendix.

10.   Important differential diagnoses include carcinoma of the caecum, Crohn's disease, right ovarian cyst, a very low enlarged gall-bladdder, or low kidney.

11.   Important differential diagnoses of appendicitis are mesenteric adenitis, right tubal or ovarian pathology (for example salpingitis, ruptured follicular cyst), acute cholecystitis, urinary tract infection, gastroenteritis, terminal ileitis, carcinoma of the caecum.

12.   In early pregnancy there is a considerable risk of abortion, later in pregnancy the appendix may be pushed laterally and towards the right hypochondrium, making diagnosis difficult.

13.   When it is strongly considered that other pathology may be present.

14.   Peritonitis, pelvic abscess, sterility, subphrenic abscess, portal pyaemia and septicaemia.

15.   The appendix of a child contains numerous lymph follicles and lymphoid tissue. In the elderly the lumen is frequently obliterated by fibrous tissue.

16.   15 per cent.

17.   About 60 per cent.

18.   Carcinoid tumour.

19.   Right hemicolectomy.

20.   A rare condition in which the peritoneal cavity becomes filled with masses of gelatinous pseudomucin sometimes years after rupture or removal of an ovarian cyst or mucocoele of the appendix.

12 APPENDIX

1.   *The common positions for the appendix are*:

(a)   Retro-ileal
(b)   Retrocaecal
(c)   Anti-ileal
(d)   Pelvic
(e)   Paracaecal

2.   *The following symptoms are commonly found in acute appendicitis in adults*:

(a)   Anorexia
(b)   Repeated vomiting
(c)   Aching joints
(d)   Diarrhoea

(e)   Generalised colic

3.   *The following signs are commonly found in acute appendicitis*:

(a)   Fever greater than 39 °C
(b)   Guarding in the right iliac fossa
(c)   Rectal tenderness high on the right
(d)   Reduced eyeball tension

(e)   Silent bowel sounds

4.   *In the investigation of appendicitis, the following are common*:

(a)   Fluid level, right iliac fossa on erect abdominal X-ray
(b)   Lymphocytosis
(c)   Neutrophil leucocytosis
(d)   Marginally raised serum amylase
(e)   Hyponatraemia

5.   *In appendicitis in children the following features are more common than in adults*:

(a)   Bleeding *per rectum*
(b)   Diarrhoea
(c)   Signs of peritonitis
(d)   Fever over 38 °C
(e)   Repeated vomiting

Target scores U.G. 15, P.G. 20

1. (a) F
   (b) T Three-quarters are retrocaecal
   (c) F
   (d) T One-fifth are pelvic
   (e) F

2. (a) T If a patient feels hungry he rarely has appendicitis
   (b) F Multiple vomits suggest a different cause of pain
   (c) F
   (d) F This is uncommon in adults, although may occur in a pelvic or retro-ileal appendicitis
   (e) F

3. (a) F A high fever is unusual in appendicitis
   (b) T
   (c) T
   (d) F This is only common in ill patients, for example with generalised peritonitis
   (e) F This sign of generalised peritonitis is uncommon in acute appendicitis

4. (a) F A fluid level is not a common feature
   (b) F ⎫
   (c) T ⎬ Neutrophil leucocytosis is usual
   (d) F ⎭
   (e) F This is rare without dehydration and repeated vomiting

5. (a) F
   (b) T Diarrhoea is not unusual in children with appendicitis
   (c) T Perforation is commoner in children
   (d) T The temperature tends to be higher in children
   (e) T Repeated vomiting is more common in children

1.   What is the commonest cause of complete large-bowel obstruction?   (1)
2.   What is the commonest cause of a large-bowel fistula?   (1)
3.   What is the commonest site for carcinoma of the colon?   (1)
4.   What is the medical treatment of uncomplicated diverticular disease?   (1)

5.   What is the likely aetiology of diverticular disease?   (1)

6.   Name three complications of diverticular disease.   (1)

7.   What is the treatment of irritable colon syndrome?   (1)

8.   How does the presentation differ between carcinoma of the caecum and carcinoma of the sigmoid?   (2)

9.   Name the commonest cause of massive bleeding from the large bowel in an adult.   (2)
10.   Name two indications for colonoscopy.   (2)

11.   Name two drugs useful in the management of ulcerative colitis.   (2)

12.   Name two features that help distinguish colonic Crohn's disease from ulcerative colitis on X-ray.   (2)

13.   Name two non-intestinal medical complications of ulcerative colitis.   (2)

14.   What is the aetiology of Hirschsprung's disease?   (2)
15.   Name a conservative operation for diverticular disease.   (3)

16.   What are the indications for colectomy in ulcerative colitis?   (3)

17.   What are the clinical features that distinguish acquired megacolon from Hirschsprung's disease?   (3)

18.   What is the management of a sigmoid volvulus?   (3)

19.   What is the treatment of familial adenomatous polyposis coli?   (3)
20.   What is the commonest site of ischaemic colitis?   (3)

Target scores U.G. 20, P.G. 29, max. 39

1.   Carcinoma of the colon.
2.   Diverticular disease.
3.   Sigmoid colon.
4.   High-residue diet, added bran, bulk laxatives, such as Normacol, antispas-
modics, for example dicyclomine.
5.   Epidemiological studies suggest that the low-fibre and low-bulk diets of
developed countries predispose to viscid, low-bulk faeces, which stimulates high
intracolonic pressures resulting in pulsion diverticula.
6.   Complications include acute diverticulitis, perforation, pericolic abscess,
fistula formation, intestinal obstruction and haemorrhage.
7.   Increasing roughage, bulk laxatives and antispasmodic drugs. Diazepam
occasionally useful.
8.   Caecal carcinoma frequently presents with anaemia, right iliac fossa pain
and a mass. Carcinoma of the sigmoid presents with change of bowel habit, rectal
bleeding, and occasionally obstruction.
9.   Diverticular disease.

10.   Common indications for colonoscopy are strictures and filling defects seen
on barium enema but beyond the reach of a sigmoidoscope. It is also a useful technique for determining the extent of inflammatory disease of the large bowel and removing colonic polyps.
11.   Codeine phosphate, salazopyrin, steroid enemata, oral prednisone, intra-
muscular ACTH.
12.   Features that help distinguish Crohn's disease from ulcerative colitis are that
the former may be associated with small-bowel lesions, may involve just one segment
of the colon sparing the rectum. The mucosa may show a cobblestone appearance.
13.   Non-colonic complications of ulcerative colitis include anaemia, iritis, polyarthritis, skin manifestations such as erythema nodosum and pyoderma gangrenosum,
cirrhosis of the liver.
14.   Congenital absence of ganglia in Auerbach's and Meissner's plexuses.
15.   Two operations described are sigmoid myotomy and transverse taenia-
myotomy.
16.   Failure of medical treatment (chronicity or fulminating attack), suspicion of
malignant change, severe systemic complications.
17.   Constipation is present from birth in Hirschsprung's disease, usually starts
later in acquired megacolon. In the latter condition rectal examination shows impaction with faeces, whereas in Hirschsprung's disease there is usually an empty segment
except in the very low cases.
18.   If there are no signs of peritonitis one may attempt to deflate the hugely
distended loop by inserting a lubricated rectal tube through a sigmoidoscope. If this
fails laparotomy after correction of fluid and electrolyte depletion and excision of
the redundant loop after untwisting. A temporary colostomy is wise.
19.   Total colectomy in early adult life. Relatives should be investigated.
20.   Splenic flexure.

1.   *A large-bowel stricture may be due to*:

(a)   Gluten enteropathy
(b)   Ischaemic colitis
(c)   Diverticulitis
(d)   Crohn's disease
(e)   Plummer—Vinson syndrome

2.   *The following are common presentations of carcinoma of the caecum*:

(a)   Anaemia
(b)   Mass in right iliac fossa
(c)   Bright red bleeding *per rectum*
(d)   Large-bowel obstruction

(e)   Change in bowel habit

3.   *There is an increased incidence of colonic carcinoma in*:

(a)   Juvenile polyps
(b)   Hirschsprung's disease
(c)   Ulcerative colitis

(d)   Peutz—Jeghers syndrome

(e)   Familial polyposis coli

4.   *The extracolonic manifestations of ulcerative colitis include*:

(a)   Pyoderma gangrenosum
(b)   Arthritis
(c)   Sclerosing cholangitis
(d)   Erythema nodosum
(e)   Otosclerosis

5.   *Diverticular disease*:

(a)   Is frequently asymptomatic
(b)   May give rise to pneumaturia
(c)   Should be treated with low-residue diet
(d)   Most commonly affects the transverse colon
(e)   Is commonly associated with mucosal ulceration

Target scores U.G. 14, P.G. 19

1. (a) F   Although rarely a small bowel lymphosarcoma can occur
   (b) T   Particularly in the splenic flexure
   (c) T   As a cause of narrowing this is second only to carcinoma
   (d) T   Crohn's disease often progresses to stricture formation
   (e) F   This is an oesophageal post-cricoid web in anaemia

2. (a) T ⎫
   (b) T ⎬ These are both common presentations
   (c) F   The bleeding is usually dark if it occurs
   (d) F   Caecal carcinoma rarely obstructs and then produces small-bowel
            obstruction
   (e) T   Either loose motions or constipation

3. (a) F   These are benign lesions
   (b) F
   (c) T   Without colectomy, some 30 per cent of total colitics may go on to
            malignant change
   (d) F   There is no increased incidence of malignant disease with these
            intestinal hamartomas
   (e) T   Malignant change is almost universal unless prophylactic colectomy is
            performed

4. (a) T
   (b) T   Usually affecting multiple joints
   (c) T   Though a rare complication
   (d) T
   (e) F   There is no association

5. (a) T   Only a minority of patients with diverticulosis present to their doctors
   (b) T   Diverticular disease is the commonest cause of a vesicocolic fistula
   (c) F   High-residue diets are indicated
   (d) F   The sigmoid is commonest
   (e) F   Mucosal lesions do not occur apart from haemorrhage

1.   Name four causes of bleeding *per rectum*.   (1)

2.   Name three ways to treat haemorrhoids.   (1)

3.   What is the usual operation for carcinoma of the lower half of the
rectum?   (1)

4.   What is the commonest cause of severe anal pain on defaecation?   (1)

5.   What are first-, second- and third-degree haemorrhoids?   (1)

6.   What is the commonest site for an anal fissure?   (1)

7.   What is the conservative treatment of an anal fissure?   (2)

8.   What is the surgical operation for the treatment of an anal fissure?   (2)

9.   What is a 'sentinel pile'?   (2)

10.   Name four causes of pruritus ani.   (2)

11.   Name two operations for complete rectal prolapse.   (2)

12.   What are the two commonest forms of abscess in the anorectal region?   (2)

13.   What is the usual management of a fistula in ano?   (2)

14.   Name two causes of secondary haemorrhoids.   (2)

15.   What is the usual cause of thrombosed haemorrhoids?   (2)

16.   What is the difference between partial and complete rectal prolapse?   (3)

17.   What is the Duke method of staging carcinoma of the rectum?   (3)

18.   What are the three usual sites of internal haemorrhoids?   (3)

19.   What is proctalgia fugax?   (3)

20.   Name three tumours of the anus.   (3)

Target scores U.G. 20, P.G. 30, max. 39

1.   Among the important causes are haemorrhoids and fissure, polyps and carcinoma of the large bowel, diverticular disease, ulcerative colitis, ischaemic colitis and bleeding disorders.

2.   Lord's anal dilatation, injection of phenol in oil, Baron's rubber band ligation, haemorrhoidectomy and cryosurgery.

3.   Abdominoperineal excision of rectum.

4.   Anal fissure (haemorrhoids are commoner but only produce severe pain when thrombosis follows prolapse).

5.   First degree = bleeding but no prolapse; second degree = prolapse on defaecation; third degree = continual prolapse of haemorrhoids.

6.   Midline posteriorly.

7.   Local anaesthetic jelly and anal dilator, or manual dilatation of anus under anaesthetic.

8.   Internal sphincterotomy (either lateral or combined with fissurectomy).

9.   An oedematous tag at the distal end of an anal fissure.

10.   Numerous causes including (1) local causes such as leakage of mucus from haemorrhoids, proctitis, etc., threadworms; (2) skin diseases such as fungal infections; (3) general causes of pruritus, for example diabetes, jaundice; (4) self-perpetuating — excessive sweating, lack of cleanliness, trauma from continuous scratching.

11.   The list of numerous procedures includes rectosigmoidectomy, anterior resection, Thiersch wire, Ivalon sponge rectopexy.

12.   The commonest is peri-anal, next is ischiorectal.

13.   The complete laying open of the fistula tract, allowing secondary healing.

14.   Pregnancy, proximal carcinoma, portal hypertension.

15.   Precipitating cause for thrombosed haemorrhoids is frequently sudden prolapse through a tight external sphincter.

16.   A partial rectal prolapse contains mucosa only; a complete rectal prolapse contains the full thickness of the rectal wall.

17.   Stage A: growth is confined to the wall of the rectum. Stage B: tumour has penetrated rectal wall to involve pararectal tissue. Stage C: lymphatic metastases are present. A stage D (= distant metastases) is commonly added to the original classification.

18.   With the patient in the lithotomy position, so that 12 o'clock is midline anteriorly, the common sites of primary haemorrhoids are at 3, 7 and 11 o'clock.

19.   Fleeting episodes of severe rectal pain, possibly due to spasm in the levator ani muscles.

20.   Tumours include squamous cell carcinoma, adenocarcinoma of the rectum invading anus, malignant melanoma, basal cell carcinoma, lymphoma.

14 ANORECTUM

1.   *Haemorrhoids*:

(a)   Are commoner in developed countries
(b)   Drain into the internal iliac veins
(c)   May rarely be secondary to portal hypertension
(d)   Usually cause dark venous bleeding

(e)   May start in late pregnancy

2.   *In the treatment of haemorrhoids*:

(a)   Surgery is usually required
(b)   Rubber-band ligation is useful for external piles
(c)   Injection is into the draining haemorrhoidal veins

(d)   Cryosurgery is ineffective
(e)   Manual dilatation of the anus does not stop bleeding from piles

3.   *A fissure in ano*:

(a)   May require internal sphincterotomy
(b)   Is commonest in the midline posteriorly
(c)   May complicate Crohn's disease

(d)   May show internal sphincter in the fissure base

(e)   Is commonly associated with a fistula in ano

4.   *Carcinoma of the rectum*:

(a)   Is more common in males
(b)   Commonly presents with sacral pain
(c)   Always requires a colostomy in management
(d)   Is usually a squamous cell carcinoma
(e)   Blood spread is usually to the liver

5.   *Fistulas in ano*:

(a)   Rarely resolve spontaneously
(b)   Usually involve the rectum above the anorectal ring
(c)   Excision and suture is usually curative
(d)   Are related to anal gland infection
(e)   Are frequently secondary to anorectal abscesses

Target scores U.G. 10, P.G. 15

1. (a)   T   Haemorrhoids are related to a fibre-depleted diet
   (b)   F   Drainage of haemorrhoidal veins is into the portal system
   (c)   T
   (d)   F   Venous bleeding is rare — the bright blood comes from rich arteriolar
             blood in the anal cushions
   (e)   T   Secondary to compression of the draining veins

2. (a)   F   Haemorrhoidectomy is unnecessary in most cases
   (b)   F   This technique is only useful in internal haemorrhoids
   (c)   F   Unlike varicose veins, the injection is into the submucosa around the
             vein pedicle and not into the vein
   (d)   F   This is an acceptable alternative to excision
   (e)   F   Dilatation under anaesthetic relieves haemorrhoidal bleeding

3. (a)   T   If it persists in spite of conservative measures
   (b)   T   This is the commonest site
   (c)   T   Some 30 per cent of patients with Crohn's disease develop anal
             complications
   (d)   T   A chronic anal fissure often exposes the transverse fibres of the inter-
             nal sphincter
   (e)   F   They are uncommonly associated

4. (a)   T
   (b)   F   This is a sign of advanced local disease
   (c)   F   Patients with high tumours can have conservation of the anal canal
   (d)   F   Most cases are adenocarcinomas
   (e)   T

5. (a)   T   Most patients require surgery
   (b)   F   Fortunately high fistulas are rare
   (c)   F   Most cases require healing by second intention
   (d)   T   This seems to be the underlying origin of fistulas in ano
   (e)   T   Many fistulas follow abscess formation

1.   Name three causes of extrahepatic obstructive jaundice in adults.   (1)

2.   Name three causes of hepatocellular jaundice.   (1)

3.   Name two causes of haemolytic jaundice.   (1)

4.   What is the commonest presentation of portal hypertension?   (1)
5.   Name two causes of portal hypertension.   (2)

6.   What are the common sites of portosystemic venous anastomoses in portal hypertension?   (2)

7.   What is a caput medusae?   (2)
8.   Name three clinical features of hepatic failure.   (2)

9.   Name three causes of cirrhosis.   (2)

10.   Name two causes of cysts in the liver.   (2)
11.   What is a Riedel's lobe?   (2)

12.   What is the purpose of a Casoni test?   (2)
13.   What is a Senstaken tube?   (2)

14.   Name two types of primary liver tumour.   (3)
15.   What is leptospirosis?   (3)

16.   Name two causes of portal pyaemia.   (3)

17.   What is an alternative name for Kinnier Wilson's disease?   (3)
18.   What is the value of an alpha-fetoprotein estimation in a patient with liver disease?   (3)
19.   What is the commonest cause of cirrhosis in the tropics?   (3)
20.   What is the Budd—Chiari syndrome?   (3)

Target scores U.G. 19, P.G. 29, max. 43

1.　　　Important causes are gall-stones, carcinoma of the pancreas, carcinoma of the gall-bladder and bile ducts, biliary stricture, carcinoma of the ampulla of Vater, carcinoma of the duodenum, sclerosing cholangitis.

2.　　　Examples are infective hepatitis, glandular fever, leptospirosis, drugs cirrhosis, liver poisons (for example carbon tetrachloride), primary and secondary liver tumours.

3.　　　Examples are congenital spherocytosis, pernicious anaemia, sickle-cell disease, thalassaemia, autoimmune haemolysis, incompatible blood transfusion.

4.　　　Bleeding oesophageal varices.

5.　　　Cirrhosis of the liver, obliteration of the portal vein from umbilical sepsis in babies, Budd—Chiari syndrome.

6.　　　Between the left gastric vein and the oesophageal veins, between the umbilical vein and superior and inferior epigastric veins, between the superior and middle haemorrhoidal veins, between diaphragmatic and retroperitoneal veins and the portal system.

7.　　　The appearance of the dilated peri-umbilical veins in portal hypertension.

8.　　　The many features include spider naevi, liver palms, flapping tremor, mental changes, hepatic coma, testicular atrophy, gynaecomastia and amenorrhoea, leukonychia, foetor, jaundice, ascites and leg oedema.

9.　　　Causes include alcoholism, nutritional (protein deficiency), primary and secondary biliary cirrhosis, severe congestive failure, post hepatitis, poisons, Wilson's disease, haemochromatosis.

10.　　　Congenital solitary cyst, polycystic disease of the liver and hydatid disease.

11.　　　Congenitally enlarged right lobe of the liver which may project down into the right iliac fossa.

12.　　　Detection of hydatid disease (complement fixation test now available).

13.　　　Triple lumen tube used to compress oesophageal varices after massive haematemesis.

14.　　　Hepatoma, cholangiocarcinoma.

15.　　　Weil's disease or 'sewer-workers' disease', a rare infective hepatocellular jaundice transmitted by rats.

16.　　　Any severe intra-abdominal infection draining into the portal system, the commonest causes being appendicitis and diverticular disease (acute diverticulitis, perforated diverticulum).

17.　　　Hepatolenticular degeneration.

18.　　　This test is positive in **60** per cent of cases of hepatoma.

19.　　　Schistosomiasis.

20.　　　Obstruction to the hepatic veins causing usually severe hepatic insufficiency and portal hypertension. The underlying cause is usually a neoplasm or hepatic vein thrombosis.

1.   *In a patient with obstructive jaundice, a diagnosis of gall-stones would be supported by the following features*:

(a)   Fluctuating jaundice
(b)   Rigors
(c)   Palpable gall-bladder
(d)   Age below 50

(e)   Very pale stools

2.   *The following clinical features may be present portal hypertension*:

(a)   Shifting dullness
(b)   Spider naevi
(c)   Onychogryphosis
(d)   Malar flushing
(e)   Succussion splash

3.   *A diagnosis of hydatid disease would be supported by*:

(a)   A solitary large transonic area on ultrasound of the liver
(b)   Passage of tape-worm fragments in the stools
(c)   Calcification ring plain film liver area
(d)   Positive Kveim test
(e)   Patient has recently migrated from Australia

4.   *The following features of liver failure are common*:

(a)   Fine tremor of hands
(b)   Testicular atrophy
(c)   Palmar erythema
(d)   Bleeding tendency

(e)   Campbell de Morgan spots

5.   *In the treatment of liver failure the following measures are useful*:

(a)   High protein diet
(b)   Magnesium sulphate
(c)   Intravenous glucose
(d)   Neomycin
(e)   Ammonium chloride

Target scores U.G. 13, P.G. 18

1. (a) T   This suggests intermittent obstruction
   (b) T   Rigors are common with cholangitis secondary to stones
   (c) F   Not if Courvoisier's law is right!
   (d) T   Apart from drugs and stones, other causes of cholestasis are uncommon below 50
   (e) F   Pale stools can occur from other causes

2. (a) T   From ascites
   (b) T
   (c) F   This is a disorder of the hallux nail
   (d) F ⎫
   (e) F ⎬ There is no association with these

3. (a) T   This would suggest a liver cyst
   (b) F   The dog gets the tape worm!
   (c) T   This is a common feature of hydatid cysts
   (d) F   This is positive in sarcoid — the Casoni test is hydatid
   (e) T   Hydatid is commoner in Australia

4. (a) F   Coarse flapping tremor is usual
   (b) T
   (c) T   'Liver palms'
   (d) T   Due to prolonged prothrombin time and deficiency of other clotting factors
   (e) F   There is no association

5. (a) F   Low-protein diet indicated
   (b) T   Useful for reducing colonic flora
   (c) T
   (d) T   As for (b)
   (e) F

1.   Name four important constituents of bile.   (1)

2.   What is cholecystokinin?   (1)

3.   Name three congenital abnormalities of the biliary tree.   (1)

4.   Name three types of gall-stones.   (1)
5.   Name three special X-ray procedures to demonstrate the biliary tree.   (1)

6.   Give two complications of acute cholecystitis.   (1)

7.   Give three complications of cholecystectomy.   (1)

8.   Name a medical condition associated with a high incidence of gall-stones.   (2)
9.   What percentage of gall-stones are visible on a plain X-ray?   (2)
10.   What is the commonest presentation of choledocholithiasis?   (2)
11.   What is Courvoisier's Law?   (2)
12.   Which bile acid taken orally has been shown to dissolve gall-stones?   (2)
13.   What is the usual precipitating cause of acute cholecystitis?   (2)
14.   What is a mucocele of the gall-bladder; where else in the body may a mucocele be found?   (3)
15.   What is gall-stone ileus?   (3)

16.   What is an alternative name for a 'strawberry gall-bladder'?   (3)
17.   What happens to the bile acid pool in gall-stone disease?   (3)
18.   What is a choledochus cyst and how does it present?   (3)

19.   What is sclerosing cholangitis?   (3)

20.   What is the cause of 'intermittent hepatic fever of Charcot'?   (3)

Target scores U.G. 18, P.G. 28, max. 40

1.   Bile salts, bile pigments, cholesterol, other lipids especially phospholipids, lecithin, triglycerides and free fatty acids, proteins including nucleoproteins, mucin, alkaline phosphatase, inorganic salts and water.

2,   Cholecystokinin is a hormone produced by the mucosa of the duodenum in response to food, especially fat. It induces gall-bladder contraction and probably relaxation of the sphincter of Oddi.

3.   Many anomalies such as congenital absence, reduplication, atresia of the ducts, long mesentery of the gall-bladder, absent cystic duct, long cystic duct opening directly into duodenum, plus numerous anomalies of the arterial supply.

4.   Mixed, cholesterol, pigment.

5.   Cholecystogram, intravenous cholangiogram, operative cholangiogram, T-tube cholangiogram, percutaneous transhepatic cholangiography, endoscopic retrograde cholangiogram.

6.   Complications include empyema of the gall-bladder, gangrene, perforation, cholecystoduodenal fistula, septicaemia, subphrenic abscess.

7.   Local complications include haemorrhage, infection, subphrenic abscess, biliary leak, damage to hepatic artery and biliary tree. General complications: chest infection, deep vein thrombosis, pulmonary embolism.

8.   Haemolytic anaemia, hypercholesterolaemia.

9.   Ten per cent.

10.   Jaundice: may be fluctuating and associated with pain.

11.   In the presence of jaundice a palpable gall-bladder is not due to gall-stones.

12.   Chenodeoxycholic acid.

13.   Obstruction of the cystic duct by a gall-stone in Hartmann's pouch.

14.   A mucocele occurs when the gall-bladder continues to produce mucus in the presence of outlet obstruction, but without infection or a thick fibrotic wall. A mucocele also occurs in the appendix.

15.   Intestinal obstruction from a large gall-stone in the terminal ileum; classically the stone erodes through the gall-bladder into the duodenum during an attack of cholecystitis.

16.   Cholesterosis.

17.   Patients with gall-stone disease have a reduced bile-salt pool.

18.   Congenital dilatation of the common bile duct, presenting with attacks of cholangitis, right upper-quadrant pain and a mass in young adults.

19.   Rare chronic disease characterised by multiple idiopathic strictures of the intra- and extrahepatic bile ducts. A quarter of cases are associated with ulcerative colitis.

20.   Cholangitis, secondary to bile-duct stones.

1.   *The following conditions predispose to the development of gall-stones:*

(a)   Hyperparathyroidism
(b)   Ileal resection
(c)   Thalassaemia
(d)   Hypercholesterolaemia
(e)   Splenectomy

2.   *The following substances are common constituents of gall-stones:*

(a)   Calcium phosphate
(b)   Calcium bilirubinate
(c)   Xanthine
(d)   Cystine
(e)   Purine

3.   *Gall-stones clinically may present with:*

(a)   Chance finding on plain X-ray of abdomen
(b)   Acute pancreatitis
(c)   Right upper-quadrant mass
(d)   Rigor with jaundice
(e)   Intestinal obstruction

4.   *'White bile' in the gall-bladder:*

(a)   Is mainly composed of mucus
(b)   Is usually secondary to adenomyosis of the gall-bladder
(c)   Is associated with blockage of the cystic duct
(d)   Is nearly always associated with jaundice
(e)   Is due to inflammatory exudate

5.   *Carcinoma of the gall-bladder:*

(a)   Is rare
(b)   Is commoner in men
(c)   Is nearly always associated with gall-stones
(d)   A palpable mass is usual
(e)   Liver scan is diagnostic

Target scores U.G. 11, P.G. 16

1. (a)   F   Renal stones are common, however
   (b)   T   Due to interruption of enterohepatic circulation of bile salts
   (c)   T   Any haemolytic anaemia can produce pigment stones
   (d)   T   Due to increased cholesterol excretion
   (e)   F   There is no increased incidence of stones after splenectomy

2. (a)   F
   (b)   T   This is the common constituent apart from cholesterol
   (c)   F
   (d)   F
   (e)   F

3. (a)   T   Gall-stones are often symptomless, some 10 per cent calcify
   (b)   T   Some 50 per cent of cases now are associated with gall-stone disease
   (c)   T   Due to mucocoele or empyema
   (d)   T   Due to cholangitis with a stone in the common bile duct
   (e)   T   Rarely a large gall-stone erodes into the gut and obstructs the terminal ileum

4. (a)   T ⎫
   (b)   F ⎬ 'White bile' occurs either in the completely obstructed gall-bladder or
   (c)   T ⎨ less commonly in severe prolonged obstructive jaundice
   (d)   F ⎭
   (e)   F

5. (a)   T
   (b)   F   Like all biliary problems, the fairer sex predominates!
   (c)   T   It is very rare without cholecystitis
   (d)   T
   (e)   F   Liver scan shows a large cold area but this feature may occur in primary or secondary liver tumours

1.   Name two enzymes and two hormones produced by the pancreas.   (1)

2.   Name a congenital anomaly of the pancreas.   (1)
3.   Name three aetiological factors in acute pancreatitis.   (2)

4.   What is the mortality of acute pancreatitis?   (2)
5.   What percentage of patients with acute pancreatitis have gall-stones?   (2)
6.   What is the treatment of acute pancreatitis?   (2)

7.   Name three complications of pancreatitis.   (2)

8.   Name two common presentations of chronic pancreatitis.   (2)

9.   What feature may be seen on a plain abdominal X-ray in chronic
pancreatitis?   (2)
10.   What is the treatment of a pseudocyst of the pancreas?   (3)

11.   What is the commonest site of a carcinoma of the pancreas?   (3)
12.   What special investigations may be of value in establishing the diagnosis
of carcinoma of the pancreas?   (3)

13.   What is the commonest treatment for carcinoma of the head of the
pancreas?   (3)
14.   Name two hormones that may be produced in excess by islet-cell
tumours.   (3)
15.   What is the Zollinger—Ellison syndrome and its cause?   (3)

16.   Name two types of true cysts of the pancreas.   (3)

17.   What does the abbreviation ERCP stand for?   (3)
18.   What is Grey Turner's sign?   (3)
19.   What is Whipple's triad?   (3)

20.   What is Whipple's operation?   (3)

Target scores U.G. 21, P.G. 31, max. 49

1.   Enzymes: proteolytic — trypsin, chymotrypsin (and precursors), procarbo-xypeptidase, elastase; other — amylase, lipase, nucleases. Hormones: insulin, glucagon.

2.   Annular pancreas, heterotopic pancreas, congenital cysts.

3.   Known causes and associations include gall-stones, alcoholism, trauma or operation, mumps, malignant hypertension, polyarteritis nodosa, hypercalcaemia.

4.   10—15 per cent.

5.   In England and Wales 40—50 per cent.

6.   Analgesia, correction of hypovolaemia and hypocalcaemia, nasogastric aspiration, possibly aprotinin (Trasylol) and glucagon.

7.   Early complications include hypovolaemia, hypocalcaemia, hypoxia, renal failure. Late complications include pseudocyst, pancreatic abscess, subphrenic abscess.

8.   The two common presentations are chronic back pain and steatorrhoea. Less common presentations are diabetes and obstructive jaundice.

9.   Calcification in the pancreas.

10.   Internal drainage of the pseudocyst, usually by creating an opening between the cyst and the posterior wall of the stomach.

11.   75 per cent occur in the head of the pancreas.

12.   Investigations that may be of use include hypotonic duodenography, pancreatic scanning, endoscopic retrograde pancreatography, secretin—pancreazymin stimulation test with duodenal intubation, cytology, pancreatic juice.

13.   As most cases are inoperable at laparotomy, the commonest treatment is biliary bypass, usually cholecystojejunostomy.

14.   Insulin, glucagon, gastrin, secretin, vasoactive intestinal peptide.

15.   The Zollinger—Ellison syndrome is characterised by intractable recurrent peptic ulceration and frequent diarrhoea associated with a high circulating gastrin level. Most cases are associated with an alpha-cell tumour of the pancreas. Occasionally G-cell hyperplasia of the stomach is found.

16.   Fibrocystic disease, congenital cystic disease, cystadenomas, cystadeno-carcinomas.

17.   Endoscopic retrograde cholangiopancreatography.

18.   Discoloration in the loin secondary to acute pancreatitis.

19.   Three features that confirm the diagnosis of an insulinoma: (1) attacks induced by starvation; (2) hypoglycaemia demonstrated during an attack; (3) relief of an attack by sugar ingestion or infusion.

20.   Pancreaticoduodenectomy.

1.   *The following may be associated with an attack of acute pancreatitis:*

(a)   Carcinoma of the pancreas
(b)   Alcohol ingestion
(c)   Hypercalcaemia

(d)   Hypoglycaemia
(e)   Hypersecretion of glucagon

2.   *The clinical features of acute pancreatitis commonly include:*

(a)   Hypertension
(b)   Absent bowel sounds
(c)   Severe back pain
(d)   Reduced liver dullness
(e)   Fluid thrill

3.   *The following may be of value in the treatment of acute pancreatitis:*

(a)   Morphine

(b)   Aprotinin

(c)   Glucagon

(d)   Insulin

(e)   Calcium gluconate

4.   *Pseudocyst of the pancreas:*

(a)   May follow pancreatic trauma
(b)   Is lined by columnar epithelium

(c)   May undergo torsion
(d)   Requires external drainage
(e)   May be diagnosed by ultrasound

5.   *Carcinoma of the pancreas:*

(a)   Commonly arises in the islet cells
(b)   Is more common in males
(c)   Is usually inoperable
(d)   Has a higher incidence among diabetics
(e)   May have associated thrombophlebitis migrans

Target scores U.G. 11, P.G. 17

1. (a) T   A carcinoma can give rise to distal obstruction and pancreatitis
   (b) T   An attack may follow alcohol ingestion
   (c) T   There is an increased incidence of pancreatitis in hypercalcaemic states such as hyperparathyroidism
   (d) F ⎫
   (e) F ⎭ There is no association with these

2. (a) F   Hypotension is common
   (b) T
   (c) T   Epigastric pain radiating to the back is characteristic
   (d) F
   (e) F   There is rarely sufficient free fluid to demonstrate this sign

3. (a) F   It is generally accepted that this drug should be avoided because of spasm of the sphincter of Oddi
   (b) T   There is some evidence that Trasylol reduces mortality over the age of 50
   (c) T   There is evidence that glucagon relieves pain and reduces exocrine secretion
   (d) F   Although some patients develop transient glycosuria, insulin is not required
   (e) T   Fat necrosis leads to hypocalcaemia in severe cases

4. (a) T   Injury or acute pancreatitis
   (b) F   A pseudocyst of the pancreas is contained in the lesser sac of peritoneum
   (c) F   This is obviously impossible
   (d) F   This would usually cause a pancreatic fistula
   (e) T   Ultrasound will demonstrate a cystic lesion behind the stomach

5. (a) F   Islet cell malignancies are rare
   (b) T
   (c) T
   (d) T
   (e) T   Classically this is 'Trousseau's sign'

1.   Name two functions of the spleen.   (1)

2.   What is the commonest indication for splenectomy?   (1)
3.   What happens to the platelet count after splenectomy?   (1)
4.   Name an important site of referred pain in a patient with a ruptured
spleen?   (1)
5.   Name three causes of splenomegaly.   (2)

6.   Name two medical conditions where splenectomy is commonly
indicated.   (2)
7.   Name two conditions that may be mistaken for an enlarged spleen.   (2)

8.   What is the preparation for surgery of a patient with idiopathic thrombocytopenic purpura?   (2)
9.   How does surgery benefit a patient with idiopathic thrombocytopenic
purpura?   (2)
10.   What are the features of hypersplenism?   (2)
11.   Name a condition where there is a high incidence of gall-stones
associated with splenomegaly.   (2)
12.   Name two conditions that lead to spontaneous rupture of the spleen.   (3)

13.   Name two indications for splenectomy as part of some other operative
procedure.   (3)
14.   Name two complications not uncommon after splenectomy.   (3)

15.   What is Felty's syndrome?   (3)
16.   What is the success rate of splenectomy in idiopathic thrombocytopenic purpura?   (3)
17.   What is splenosis?   (3)

18.   Name two causes of massive enlargement of the spleen.   (3)

19.   What is the incidence of accessory spleens in patients with haemolytic
anaemia?   (3)
20.   Name a primary tumour of the spleen.   (3)

Target scores U.G. 19, P.G. 28, max. 45

1.　　　　Antibody formation, removal of damaged red cells and other particulate matter from the circulation. It may also store platelets, and in infants and adults when the bone marrow activity is grossly suppressed, the spleen may produce blood cells.

2.　　　　Trauma.

3.　　　　Usually marked increase of platelets, maximally at about three weeks.

4.　　　　To the shoulders.

5.　　　　Numerous causes including (1) infections (glandular fever, typhoid, malaria, schistosomiasis); (2) blood disorders, for example leukaemia, Hodgkin's disease, pernicious anaemia, polycythaemia, congenital spherocytosis, acquired haemolytic anaemia, thrombocytopenic purpura; (3) portal hypertension; (4) metabolic and collagen diseases (amyloid, Gaucher's disease, Still's disease).

6.　　　　Examples are haemolytic anaemia (for example spherocytosis), thrombocytopenic purpura, staging of Hodgkin's disease.

7.　　　　Enlarged kidney (for example hydronephrosis), carcinoma of the stomach, carcinoma of the splenic flexure.

8.　　　　If purpuric, patient will need steroids; if actively bleeding, patient will require platelets immediately pre-operatively.

9.　　　　Splenectomy reduces platelet breakdown.

10.　　　Large spleen associated with pancytopenia and an active bone marrow.

11.　　　Any haemolytic anaemia, particularly spherocytosis.

12.　　　Any chronic enlargement of the spleen, particularly malaria, glandular fever and leukaemia.

13.　　　Common procedures are as a part of radical excision of carcinoma of the stomach, splenorenal anastomosis, and of course accidental damage at operation.

14.　　　After splenectomy there is a high incidence of thrombo-embolism and subphrenic abscess.

15.　　　Rheumatoid arthritis, neutropenia and splenomegaly.

16.　　　65 per cent success rate.

17.　　　Rare condition when following traumatic rupture of the spleen, multiple implants of splenic tissue grow scattered throughout the peritoneal cavity.

18.　　　Chronic myeloid leukaemia, polycythaemia, portal hypertension, schistosomiasis, myelofibrosis, Gaucher's disease, malaria.

19.　　　25 per cent.

20.　　　Benign: haemangioma. Malignant: lymphosarcoma, fibrosarcoma.

1.   *The spleen commonly enlarges in*:

(a)   Crohn's disease
(b)   Hashimoto's disease
(c)   Gaucher's disease
(d)   Still's disease
(e)   Cushing's syndrome

2.   *The following features may occur in a patient with splenic rupture*:

(a)   Absence of bowel sounds
(b)   Bruising of lower ribs
(c)   Shoulder pain
(d)   Slow pulse
(e)   Low platelet count

3.   *Splenectomy is commonly indicated in*:

(a)   Acute myeloid leukaemia
(b)   Hereditary spherocytosis
(c)   Idiopathic thrombocytopenic purpura
(d)   Sickle-cell trait
(e)   Hodgkin's disease

4.   *Splenectomy may be followed by*:

(a)   Increased red cell fragility
(b)   Leucocytosis
(c)   Increased platelet count
(d)   Decreased blood viscosity
(e)   Increased incidence of thrombo-embolism

5.   *Gaucher's disease*:

(a)   May result in massive splenomegaly
(b)   Is more common in Egyptians
(c)   Is due to abnormal storage of kerosene
(d)   Is associated with anaemia
(e)   Frequently requires splenectomy

Target scores U.G. 12, P.G. 17

1. (a) F
   (b) F   This disease affects the thyroid
   (c) T   A large spleen is common
   (d) T   In association with juvenile rheumatoid arthritis
   (e) F

2. (a) T   Bowel sounds are usually reduced or absent
   (b) T   Evidence of trauma to left lower rib cage is usual
   (c) T   Referred pain to the shoulder due to blood irritating the diaphragm
   (d) F   Shock is usual
   (e) F

3. (a) F   Splenectomy does not benefit this leukaemia
   (b) T   Splenectomy increases the life span of the abnormal red cells
   (c) T   Many patients benefit from splenectomy
   (d) F
   (e) T   It is indicated for accurate staging of the disease

4. (a) F
   (b) T   Leucocytosis often lasts for several months
   (c) T   The platelets may temporarily exceed 1 million/cu mm
   (d) F   Only if the patient bleeds!
   (e) T   There is an increased risk of DVT

5. (a) T   The spleen may be enormous
   (b) F   Slavonic and Jewish races may be more prone
   (c) F   Kerasin, not kerosene!
   (d) T   Anaemia is usual
   (e) T   Mainly to get rid of the bulky abdominal mass — it does not stop the
            progress of the disease

19 KIDNEY AND URETER

1.   Name two causes of unilateral hydronephrosis.   (1)

2.   Name two causes of bilateral hydronephrosis.   (1)

3.   Name three congenital anomalies of the kidney.   (1)

4.   What is a pyeloplasty?   (1)

5.   What is an alternative name for a Wilms' tumour?   (1)
6.   What is the management of renal trauma?   (1)

7.   Name three complications of a hydronephrosis.   (1)

8.   Name four causes of renal calculi.   (2)

9.   What are three common types of urinary calculi?   (2)

10.   What percentage of urinary calculi presenting to a surgeon are visible on
a plain abdominal X-ray?   (2)
11.   What is the significance of a sterile acid pyuria?   (2)
12.   What is the common age and presentation of a Wilms' tumour?   (2)

13.   What is the treatment of a Wilms' tumour?   (2)

14.   What are the common presentations of polycystic kidneys?   (2)

15.   What is the purpose of a Dormia basket?   (2)

16.   What is the management of acute calculus anuria?   (3)

17.   At what three common sites do ureteric calculi tend to lodge?   (3)

18.   Name two types of renal stones not visible on a plain X-ray.   (3)
19.   Name two complications of a horseshoe kidney.   (3)

20.   Name three clinical presentations of a renal carcinoma.   (3)

Target scores U.G. 18, P.G. 28, max. 38

1.　　　Congenital: for example pelvi-ureteric neuromuscular incoordination or aberrant vessel, vesico-ureteric reflux, ureterocoele. Ureteric obstruction: for example stone, tumour, stricture, carcinoma of bladder.

2.　　　Congenital (as above), bladder outlet obstruction due to prostatic hypertrophy or urethral stricture, posterior urethral valves, bilateral vesico-ureteric reflux, carcinoma of the bladder or cervix.

3.　　　Examples are atresia, polycystic kidney, horseshoe kidney, pelvic kidney, double kidney, double ureter, absence, crossed ectopia.

4.　　　Operation on the pelvis and pelvi-ureteric junction to correct congenital hydronephrosis.

5.　　　Nephroblastoma.

6.　　　The vast majority can be managed conservatively. An emergency IVP should be done mainly to check function of other kidney. Renal angiography may be indicated. Rarely exploration and possible nephrectomy.

7.　　　Complications include infection possibly leading to pyonephrosis, stone formation, hypertension, reduced renal function and uraemia in severe cases.

8.　　　Factors predisposing to renal calculi are chronic stasis, chronic infection, immobilisation, hypercalcuria (for example in hyperparathyroidism, immobilisation, vitamin D intoxication, milk-alkali syndrome, sarcoidosis), excessive uric acid excretion (gout, leukaemia, polycythaemia), the presence of abnormal constituents in the urine,(for example cystinuria), medullary sponge kidney.

9.　　　Triple phosphate calculi, calcium oxalate calcium carbonate and uric acid. Rarely cystine, xanthine ammonium and sodium urate.

10.　　90 per cent.

11.　　The possibility of a tuberculous infection.

12.　　Usually children under the age of four presenting with a mass. Haematuria, occurs in about 20 per cent.

13.　　The mainstay of treatment is radical nephrectomy; chemotherapy and radiotherapy are also used.

14.　　Swelling, haematuria, loin discomfort, renal infection, hypertension, renal failure.

15.　　The cystoscopic extraction of calculi from the lowest few centimetres of the ureter.

16.　　Urgent relief of the obstruction. This may require ureteric catheterisation beyond the stone, nephrostomy, or removal of the stone.

17.　　Pelvi-ureteric junction, where the ureter crosses the pelvic brim and the intramural part of the ureter.

18.　　Uric-acid stones and amino-acid stones (for example cystine stones).

19.　　Horseshoe kidneys are predisposed to infection, hydronephrosis and stone formation, with all the complications of both.

20.　　Haematuria, clot colic, abdominal mass, loin aching, pathological fracture, anaemia, weight loss, pyrexia of unknown origin, occasionally as pulmonary metastases, acute varicocoele or polycythaemia.

1.   *A patient with blunt abdominal trauma develops haematuria*:

(a)   Urgent selective renal arteriography is indicated in most cases
(b)   The kidney should be explored
(c)   An intravenous urogram is of no value in the early stages

(d)   Cystoscopy and retrograde pyelogram gives maximum information
(e)   Surgery is rarely indicated

2.   *A patient develops renal colic. An emergency IVU*:

(a)   Is rarely informative due to gas shadows
(b)   Often shows delayed excretion on the affected side
(c)   Often shows dilution of contrast on unaffected side
(d)   Often shows urine extravasation on the affected side
(e)   May be completely normal

3.   *Vesico-ureteric reflux is adequately assessed by which of the following investigations*:

(a)   Ultrasound
(b)   Micturating cystogram

(c)   Cystoscopy
(d)   Urethrogram
(e)   Retrograde pyelography

4.   *Adenocarcinoma of the kidney*:

(a)   Is more common in men
(b)   Metastasises mainly by the renal vein
(c)   May rarely present with PUO
(d)   May present insiduously or as a loin mass
(e)   Radiotherapy is the best primary treatment

5.   *Hydronephrosis*:

(a)   Is the commonest cause of renal failure

(b)   Always produces symptoms
(c)   Usually requires retrograde pyelography to elucidate the cause
(d)   If unilateral is usually caused by a urinary calculus
(e)   Rarely requires surgical interference

Target scores U.G. 13, P.G. 18

1. (a) F }
   (b) F } In the majority of cases expectant management is satisfactory
   (c) F The IVU is useful to demonstrate a normal contralateral kidney and gives an estimate of extent of renal damage
   (d) F A retrograde pyelogram is unhelpful and may introduce infection
   (e) T

2. (a) F Delayed excretion is informative
   (b) T
   (c) F
   (d) F Renal extravasation of contrast is very rare
   (e) T

3. (a) F
   (b) T Micturating cystogram is the only method of confirming ureteric reflux
   (c) F
   (d) F
   (e) F

4. (a) T
   (b) T
   (c) T
   (d) T
   (e) F Nephrectomy is the best primary treatment in most cases

5. (a) F Chronic pyelonephritis and glomerulonephritis are much commoner causes
   (b) F A hydronephrosis may be symptom-free
   (c) F Diagnosis can nearly always be made on intravenous urography
   (d) T
   (e) F Many cases of hydronephrosis require to be relieved by some surgical procedure

1. Give three common causes of haematuria. (1)

2. Give three causes of urine retention. (1)

3. Name the commonest type of urinary diversion. (1)
4. What is the commonest organism causing acute cystitis? (1)
5. What is the standard treatment of most bladder tumours? (1)
6. What is the cause of most bladder diverticula? (2)
7. What is the classical symptom of a large bladder diverticulum? (2)
8. What are the symptoms of a bladder stone? (2)

9. What instrument is used for crushing a bladder stone? (2)
10. Name two effects of chronic bladder outlet obstruction. (2)

11. Name two indications for urinary diversion. (2)

12. Name two complications of ureteric reflux. (3)

13. What is the usual management of deeply invasive bladder cancer? (3)
14. What is the cause of a urinary leak from the umbilicus? (3)
15. Name two predisposing causes for carcinoma of the bladder. (3)

16. How may one differentiate clinically between an intraperitoneal and and an extraperitoneal rupture of the bladder? (3)

17. Give two complications of bladder diverticula. (3)
18. What dose of radiotherapy is required for radical treatment of bladder cancer? (3)
19. What is the usual treatment of severe stress incontinence? (3)
20. What is ectopia vesicae? (3)

Target scores U.G. 19, P.G. 29, max. 44

1.   Common causes are urinary-tract infection, prostatic hypertrophy, urinary calculi and tumours. Less common causes include hydronephrosis, bleeding diatheses, polycystic disease, trauma and carcinoma of prostate.

2.   Relatively common causes are benign enlargement of the prostate, carcinoma of the prostate, urethral stricture, faecal impaction, pelvic or anal surgery and some drugs (for example atropine-like group). Less common causes are bladder or urethral stone, clot retention, phimosis, neurological disorders (spinal cord lesions, for example), retroverted gravid uterus.

3.   Ileal conduit.

4.   *E. coli.*

5.   Cystodiathermy.

6.   Bladder outlet obstruction.

7.   Double micturition.

8.   Frequency, pain, particularly at the end of micturition, haematuria, intermittent interruption of the urinary stream with pain.

9.   A lithotrite.

10.   Detrusor hypertrophy, trabeculation, sacculation, diverticulum formation, eventual detrusor stretching and atonicity, dilatation of the ureters and hydronephrosis, uraemia, stone formation.

11.   Incontinence (for example spina bifida, ectopia vesicae), severe contracted bladder (chronic cystitis, tuberculosis and following cystectomy for carcinoma of the bladder).

12.   Urinary infections, hydronephrosis, stone formation, acute and chronic pyelonephritis.

13.   High-voltage radiotherapy, sometimes followed by cystectomy.

14.   A patent urachus; rarely, bladder cancer.

15.   Occupational hazards (for example in aniline-dye workers, and in the rubber industry), smoking, bladder diverticula, congenital anomalies (for example ectopia vesicae), schistosomiasis.

16.   Intraperitoneal rupture produces peritonitis and paralytic ileus. Extraperitoneal rupture produces extrasavation of urine into the pelvic connective tissue and lower abdominal wall.

17.   Infection, stone formation, malignant change, rarely rupture.

18.   6000 rads.

19.   Retropubic bladder sling.

20.   Congenital anomaly in which the bladder opens out onto the abdominal wall, associated with gross hypospadias and deficit of pubic bones.

1.   *A woman of 56 presents with haematuria. Which of the following would be the likely causes*:

(a)   Bleeding disorder
(b)   Urinary infection
(c)   Cystinuria
(d)   Bladder tumour
(e)   Cushing's syndrome

2.   *Bladder cancer may be associated with*:

(a)   *Entamoeba histolytica* infestation
(b)   Exposure to phosphorus
(c)   Bilharziasis
(d)   Working with beta-naphthylamine
(e)   Heavy smoking

3.   *Most bladder cancers*:

(a)   Present with dysuria
(b)   Are papillary
(c)   Are adenocarcinomas
(d)   Present in the 5th—6th decades
(e)   Recur after treatment

4.   *Bladder diverticula*:

(a)   Are more common in males
(b)   Are usually congenital
(c)   May obstruct the ureter
(d)   Predispose to urinary infection

(e)   May contain tumour

5.   *Chronic retention of urine*:

(a)   Is usually painful
(b)   May present with uraemia
(c)   Leads to contracted bladder
(d)   Frequently results in incontinence
(e)   Usually responds to drug therapy alone

Target scores U.G. 15, P.G. 20

1. (a)   F   This would be rare
   (b)   T   This is the commonest cause of haematuria
   (c)   F
   (d)   T   This would be the second commonest cause of haematuria at this age
   (e)   F

2. (a)   F   Hydatid has no relation to bladder cancer
   (b)   F
   (c)   T   Schistosomiasis is commonly complicated by malignant change
   (d)   T   Used in aniline-dye industry
   (e)   T   There is a statistically increased risk in heavy smokers

3. (a)   F   Dysuria is far less common than haematuria
   (b)   T
   (c)   F   Transitional cell carcinomas are commonest
   (d)   T
   (e)   T   Recurrence or new lesions are common

4. (a)   T   Due to bladder outlet obstruction
   (b)   F
   (c)   T   Hydronephrosis may occasionally be due to a large diverticulum
   (d)   T   Due to stasis of urine in the diverticulum and from the outflow obstruction
   (e)   T   Malignant change is well recognised

5. (a)   F   Pain is frequently absent
   (b)   T
   (c)   F   Atonic bladder
   (d)   T   Retention with overflow incontinence is common
   (e)   F   Drug treatment has little place in neurogenic bladder or outflow obstruction

1.   Name four symptoms common in a patient with benign enlargement of the prostate.   (1)
2.   What is the main distinction between acute retention and chronic retention from the history?   (1)
3.   What is the primary treatment of most cases of carcinoma of the prostate?   (1)
4.   How does the presentation of carcinoma of the prostate differ from benign enlargement of the prostate?   (1)
5.   How does rectal examination distinguish between benign and malignant enlargement of the prostate?   (1)

6.   What is the best method of obtaining positive histology in suspected prostatic cancer?   (2)
7.   What is the value of isotopic studies in prostatic carcinoma?   (2)

8.   What are the common sites for metastases in carcinoma of the prostate? (2)
9.   What is unusual about bony deposits from carcinoma of the prostate? (2)

10.   Name two unwanted effects of oestrogen treatment for carcinoma of the prostate.   (2)
11.   Name four complications of benign enlargement of the prostate.   (2)

12.   What is the 'surgical capsule' of the prostate?   (2)
13.   How many lobes has the enlarged prostate?   (2)
14.   Name two complications of prostatectomy.   (2)

15.   Name three methods of prostatectomy.   (3)

16.   Name two conditions that may mimic the symptoms of an enlarged prostate.   (3)
17.   What is the normal prostatic weight?   (3)
18.   What are the normal components of the prostate gland?   (3)
19.   What is the incidence of a high serum acid-phosphatase level in patients with carcinoma of the prostate?   (3)
20.   Besides oestrogen, what other treatments are of value in the management of carcinoma of the prostate?   (3)

Target scores U.G. 18, P.G. 29, max. 41

1.   Clinical features include frequency, nocturia, hesitancy, poor stream, terminal dribbling, haematuria, acute retention.

2.   Acute retention is painful and often of sudden onset. Chronic retention is painless and may be associated with overflow incontinence.

3.   Oestrogen orally (for example stilboestrol).

4.   Carcinoma tends to be in the older age group, symptoms are of quicker onset, may present with symptoms from bony metastases.

5.   A malignant prostate is characteristically hard on rectal examination. The induration may spread beyond the bounds of the prostate. There is loss of the medial and lateral sulci and the rectal mucosa may be tethered.

6.   Perineal or transrectal needle biopsy.

7.   Isotopic studies may detect bony metastases before they are visible on a plain X-ray.

8.   The commonest site is bone, particularly the lumbar spine and pelvis.

9.   Bony deposits from carcinoma of the prostate are frequently osteoblastic rather than osteolytic, hence the areas are denser on X-ray.

10.   Impotence, gynaecomastia, and increased risk of thrombo-embolism and myocardial infarction.

11.   Acute retention, chronic retention, haematuria, bilateral hydronephrosis, uraemia, urinary-tract infections.

12.   Most of the surgical capsule consists of compressed normal prostatic tissue.

13.   Three: two lateral lobes and a middle lobe.

14.   Complications include incontinence, retrograde ejaculation, impotence, urinary infection and epididymo-orchitis, stricture formation. General complications — for example chest infection, thrombo-embolism.

15.   The commonest two methods of prostatectomy are transurethral resection and retropubic prostatectomy. Others are transvesical prostatectomy and perineal prostatectomy.

16.   Urethral stricture, bladder neck obstruction (for example fibromuscular hyperplasia).

17.   20 grams.

18.   Fibrous tissue, smooth muscle, glandular tissue.

19.   50 per cent of cases have a raised serum acid phosphatase. Most of these have bone metastases.

20.   Radical prostatectomy, transurethral resection, radiotherapy, bilateral orchidectomy, corticosteroids, hypophysectomy, and local treatment for pathological fractures.

1.   *Acute prostatitis*:

(a)   Commonly leads to rigors
(b)   May be due to *Neisseria gonorrhoeae*
(c)   Presents with perineal pain and dysuria
(d)   Usually requires drainage with a resectoscope
(e)   Rectal examination reveals a hard craggy mass

2.   *Benign enlargement of the prostate*:

(a)   Is mostly due to proliferation of fibrous tissue
(b)   Rarely occurs before the age of 60
(c)   Always produces symptoms
(d)   Rarely leads to haematuria
(e)   Is the commonest cause of retention in males

3.   *The symptoms of benign prostatic enlargement*:

(a)   Are proportional to the size of the gland
(b)   Commonly include pain on micturition
(c)   Commonly include straining to micturate
(d)   Commonly include nocturnal frequency
(e)   Commonly include bilateral loin pain

4.   *In the management of a patient with benign prostatic enlargement*:

(a)   Intravenous urography should be performed on all cases
(b)   Transurethral resection has the lowest morbidity
(c)   There is no satisfactory medical treatment
(d)   Total prostatectomy gives the best results
(e)   Associated urinary infection increases the morbidity

5.   *Which of the following statements are true of carcinoma of the prostate*:

(a)   Presentation may be with back pain
(b)   Serum acid phosphatase is nearly always diagnostic

(c)   Microscopic carcinoma of the prostate is common in the elderly
(d)   Bony metastases may be sclerotic
(e)   The tumour may respond to orchidectomy

Target scores U.G. 10, P.G. 16

1. (a)   F   Rigors are uncommon
   (b)   T   The gonococcus is frequently implicated
   (c)   T   These are common symptoms
   (d)   F   Acute prostatitis responds to medical treatment
   (e)   F   The prostate is exquisitely tender on P.R.

2. (a)   F   Glandular and muscular elements are also involved
   (b)   F   Enlargement commonly starts before the age of 60
   (c)   F   Prostatic size does not correlate closely with symptoms
   (d)   F   Haematuria is not uncommon
   (e)   T

3. (a)   F   See 2(c)
   (b)   F   Unless there is a urinary infection, pain is unusual
   (c)   F   Straining rarely helps micturition in prostatic hypertrophy
   (d)   T   This is found in almost all cases with symptoms
   (e)   F   Loin pain is not a common symptom

4. (a)   T   To check upper tracts, bladder outline and emptying
   (b)   T   Open operations have a higher mortality and morbidity
   (c)   T   Though drug firms are still searching!
   (d)   F   This is never indicated in benign disease
   (e)   T

5. (a)   T   Spinal metastases at presentation are not unusual
   (b)   F   The acid phosphatase may be normal, particularly if the carcinoma is confined to the gland
   (c)   T   80 per cent of 80-year-olds
   (d)   T   Sclerotic deposits are common
   (e)   T   Regression with orchidectomy or oestrogen is common

1.   What is the commonest medical indication for circumcision?   (1)
2.   What is the commonest complication of circumcision?   (1)
3.   What is a urethrogram?   (1)

4.   What are the two common causes of a urethral stricture?   (1)
5.   What is the commonest treatment of a urethral stricture?   (1)
6.   What is a paraphimosis?   (1)

7.   What are the two methods of treatment for carcinoma of the penis?   (1)
8.   What is the probable aetiology of carcinoma of the penis?   (2)
9.   What is balanoposthitis?   (2)
10.   Name two indications for a urethroplasty.   (2)
11.   What is the commonest site for a urethral stricture?   (2)
12.   What is the difference between hypospadias and epispadias?   (2)

13.   What is priapism?   (2)
14.   What is a meatoplasty?   (3)
15.   What is an underlying cause for the development of priapism?   (3)

16.   What is the treatment of priapism?   (3)

17.   What is Peyronie's disease?   (3)

18.   What is an effective treatment for Peyronie's disease?   (3)

19.   Name a condition associated with Peyronie's disease.   (3)
20.   What is erythroplasia of Queyrat?   (3)

Target scores U.G. 18, P.G. 28, max. 40

1.   Phimosis.

2.   Haemorrhage (then infection).

3.   X-ray injection of contrast medium up the urethra, particularly to demonstrate urethral strictures, and possible urethral injury.

4.   Gonorrhoea and instrumentation.

5.   Urethral dilatation.

6.   A condition in which a tight foreskin is retracted beyond the corona and becomes irreducible.

7.   Local radiotherapy, amputation.

8.   Probably carcinogens in retained smegma.

9.   Balanitis is infection of the glans, posthitis is infection of the foreskin.

10.   Hypospadias and the treatment of urethral strictures.

11.   At the penoscrotal junction.

12.   In a hypospadias the urethra opens on the ventral surface; in an epispadias it opens on the dorsal surface of the penis.

13.   A condition in which the penis fails to become flaccid after an erection.

14.   An operation to widen a tight urethral meatus.

15.   25 per cent of cases are associated with hypercoaguability, as in leukaemia, metatastic carcinoma or sickle-cell anaemia.

16.   If the priapism fails to resolve in a few hours, aspiration of the sludged blood and lavage with anticoagulant may be tried. If this fails, an anastomosis between the saphenous vein and the corpus cavernosum or, alternatively, a spongiosus — cavernosum shunt should be done. In spite of these measures impotence is frequent.

17.   A condition in which a plaque of fibrous tissue is laid down in the corpus cavernosum.

18.   Hydrocortisone injection and therapeutic ultrasound are both recommended but unproven.

19.   Dupuytren's contracture, retroperitoneal fibrosis.

20.   Carcinoma *in situ* of the glans penis, similar to Bowen's disease of skin.

1.   *Indications for circumcision include:*

(a)   Recurrent balanoposthitis
(b)   Recurrent paraphimosis
(c)   Suspicion of carcinoma of glans penis
(d)   Hypospadias
(e)   Meatal stenosis

2.   *Rupture of the membranous urethra:*

(a)   Commonly follows falling astride a fence or similar object
(b)   Requires urgent primary suture
(c)   Frequently leads to extravasation of urine
(d)   Often presents with urethral bleeding and failure to micturate
(e)   May be treated by suprapubic drainage with subsequent urethrography

3.   *A urethral stricture:*

(a)   Is usually secondary to acute cystitis
(b)   May produce bilateral hydronephrosis
(c)   Predisposes to urinary infection
(d)   Commonly presents with haematuria
(e)   Usually requires urethroplasty

4.   *Carcinoma of the penis:*

(a)   Is more common in Jews
(b)   Is commonest in the 4th and 5th decades
(c)   Commonly starts on the shaft
(d)   Frequently ulcerates
(e)   Often presents with acute retention

5.   *In the treatment of carcinoma of the penis:*

(a)   Early growths can be satisfactorily treated by radiotherapy
(b)   Radical amputation offers the only hope of cure
(c)   Groin dissection of nodes may be necessary
(d)   Orchidectomy should be routine
(e)   Only 5 per cent of patients survive five years

Target scores U.G. 13, P.G. 18

1. (a) T This is inflammation of glans and foreskin
   (b) T This is the commonest indication for circumcision in adults
   (c) T Diagnosis may be impossible to confirm without circumcision
   (d) F The foreskin must be preserved for the plastic repair
   (e) F This requires dilatation or meatotomy

2. (a) F This would produce a rupture of the bulbar urethra
   (b) F It is a difficult area to suture
   (c) T
   (d) T This should alert one to the possibility of a ruptured urethra
   (e) T This is an acceptable alternative to 'railroading' a catheter into place

3. (a) F Urethritis or trauma
   (b) T Any chronic outflow obstruction may lead to hydronephrosis
   (c) T
   (d) F Haematuria is uncommon from stricture
   (e) F Most strictures respond to dilatation

4. (a) F It is rare in the circumcised
   (b) F It is a disease of the elderly
   (c) F It is commonest on the glans near the corona
   (d) T
   (e) F The tumour is rarely this advanced at presentation

5. (a) T And, of course, gives a better functional result than surgery
   (b) F Only if urethra and lymph nodes are involved
   (c) T If nodes are involved
   (d) F Orchidectomy has no place
   (e) F The prognosis is better than this

1. What is the commoner side of a varicocele? (1)

2. Name two common testicular tumours. (1)

3. What is the commonest site for an ectopic testis? (1)

4. What is the commonest complication of surgery for a hydrocele? (1)

5. What are the clinical features of a varicocele? (1)

6. What are the commonest lymph nodes to be affected in testicular tumours? (1)

7. What is the treatment of testicular tumours? (2)

8. Name two complications of undescended testes. (2)

9. Name four types of fluid found in cystic swellings of the scrotum. (2)

10. Name two causes of a secondary hydrocele. (2)

11. What are the clinical features of a hydrocele of the cord? (2)

12. What are the clinical features of a communicating congenital hydrocele? (2)

13. Name two indications for an orchiopexy. (2)

14. Name two indications for surgery in a varicocele. (2)

15. What is the optimum age for surgery of the undescended testicle? (2)

16. Name three clinical features that help distinguish a torsion from an epididymo-orchitis. (2)

17. What is the commonest organism to cause an epididymo-orchitis? (2)

18. Name two specific infections of the testicle. (3)

19. What is the commonest testicular tumour and the commonest age group in which it occurs? (3)

20. How can you distinguish testicular tumours on cut section? (3)

Target scores U.G. 19, P.G. 28, max. 37

1.   Left side.

2.   Seminoma, teratoma.

3.   Superficial inguinal pouch.

4.   Haematoma formation.

5.   'Bag of worms' — dilated veins which are most evident when the patient stands. A cough impulse can usually be felt.

6.   Para-aortic nodes.

7.   Radical orchidectomy plus radiotherapy.

8.   Increased risk of torsion and local trauma, infertility, liability to malignant change.

9.   Crystal-clear fluid of epididymal cysts, opalescent fluid of spermatocele, straw-coloured fluid of hydrocele, blood-stained fluid of haematocele.

10.   Acute and chronic epididymo-orchitis, gumma, testicular tumours.

11.   Soft irreducible swelling in the line of the spermatic cord, may be brilliantly transilluminable if outside external ring.

12.   Hydrocele that empties into the peritoneal cavity in horizontal position.

13.   Undescended testes, testicular torsion.

14.   Local discomfort, infertility.

15.   4—6 years old.

16.   Torsion occurs in a younger age group and tends to be of a more sudden onset; there are no associated urinary symptoms that may be present with epididymo-orchitis. In the latter condition there is tenderness of the vas and seminal vesicles on rectal examination, and pus cells may be found in the urine. Elevation of the scrotum may relieve the pain of epididymo-orchitis but will make the pain of a torsion worse.

17.   *E. coli*.

18.   Tuberculosis, syphilis.

19.   Seminoma (60 per cent) between the ages of 30 and 40.

20.   Seminoma is solid on cut section, teratoma is usually cystic — may appear like a colloid goitre.

1.   *In the clinical features of a hydrocele*:

(a)   The swelling is mainly behind the testis
(b)   The swelling usually extends to the external inguinal ring
(c)   The swelling is always brilliantly transilluminable
(d)   The testis always feels normal
(e)   The hydrocele occasionally may empty on squeezing

2.   *In patients with undescended or ectopic testes*:

(a)   Surgical treatment at puberty usually restores normal spermatogenesis
(b)   The testis is more likely to undergo torsion
(c)   Most patients respond to gonadotrophins
(d)   The best management is orchidopexy in the first year of life
(e)   Undescended testes are frequently small

3.   *Testicular torsion*:

(a)   Usually occurs in a testis that is more horizontal than normal
(b)   May be impossible to differentiate from epididymo-orchitis
(c)   Is often associated with redness of the overlying skin
(d)   In early cases should be managed conservatively by untwisting without exploration
(e)   Requires an operation on both testicles

4.   *In the diagnosis of a testicular tumour*:

(a)   Presence of pain excludes the diagnosis
(b)   Inguinal nodes are enlarged in 20 per cent of the cases
(c)   Nodularity localised to the epididymis makes the diagnosis unlikely
(d)   An associated hydrocele may occur
(e)   An abdominal mass may be palpable at presentation

5.   *Seminoma of the testes*:

(a)   Most commonly occurs below the age of 45
(b)   Is usually radioresistant
(c)   Has a better prognosis than teratoma
(d)   Blood-borne metastases are uncommon
(e)   Radical lymphadenectomy gives the best prognosis

Target scores U.G. 11, P.G. 17

1. (a) F   The tunica vaginalis envelops the front and sides of the testicle
   (b) F   It is uncommon for the hydrocele to extend this far
   (c) F   Brilliant transillumination suggests an epididymal cyst
   (d) F   Some hydroceles are secondary to testicular disease
   (e) T   Some congenital hydroceles are communicating

2. (a) F   Orchiopexy this late rarely restores normal spermatogenesis
   (b) T
   (c) F   Few maldescended testes respond to gonadotrophins
   (d) F   4–6 years
   (e) T   Undescended testes are often abnormal testes

3. (a) T   The so-called 'bell-clapper testis'
   (b) T   If in doubt, exploration is essential
   (c) F   If the history is this long the testis is probably non-viable
   (d) F   Every torsion requires early operation and fixation
   (e) T   The abnormality that predisposes to torsion is usually bilateral

4. (a) F   Some tumours present like epididymo-orchitis
   (b) F   Lymphatic spread is to para-aortic nodes unless scrotal skin is invaded
   (c) T   Paratesticular tumours are very rare
   (d) T   A small secondary hydrocele may occur
   (e) T   Involved para-aortic nodes may be palpable

5. (a) T
   (b) F   Seminoma is highly radiosensitive
   (c) T   Seminoma has a far better response to treatment
   (d) T   Blood spread is late
   (e) F   Radiotherapy is satisfactory treatment for para-aortic nodes

1.   What is the commonest cause of thoracic aneurysm?   (1)

2.   What is an alternative name for thrombo-angiitis obliterans?   (1)

3.   What is the commonest cause of fat embolism?   (1)

4.   Name a material commonly used for arterial prostheses.   (1)

5.   What is an alternative name for arterial disobliteration?   (1)

6.   What is the best method of arterial embolectomy?   (1)

7.   What is the most important part of the management of patients with
Buerger's disease?   (2)

8.   Name three emboli other than thrombus.   (2)

9.   Name two common causes of arterial emboli.   (2)

10.   What is the commonest site for a berry aneurysm?   (2)

11.   What condition predisposes to dissecting aneurysm?   (2)

12.   What is the commonest presentation of an aortic aneurysm?   (2)

13.   What is caisson disease?   (2)

14.   What percentage of claudicants go on to gangrene: 5, 10, 20 or
50 per cent?   (3)

15.   What is the mortality of a ruptured aortic aneurysm?   (3)

16.   Give two indications for a sympathectomy.   (3)

17.   Name three surgical approaches for a cervical sympathectomy.   (3)

18.   What would be the operation of choice for a patient with an ischaemic
leg and a localised common iliac stenosis due to atheroma?   (3)

19.   What are the clinical features of chronic mesenteric infarction?   (3)

20.   Name two effects of congenital arteriovenous fistula.   (3)

Target scores U.G. 18, P.G. 29, max. 41

1.   Atheroma.

2.   Buerger's disease.

3.   Long-bone fracture, usually the femur.

4.   Dacron, and Teflon.

5.   Endarterectomy.

6.   Use of a Fogarty embolectomy catheter.

7.   To stop them smoking.

8.   Air, fat, amniotic fluid, tumour, atheromatous plaques, foreign bodies and parasites.

9.   Myocardial infarction and atrial fibrillation.

10.   Circle of Willis.

11.   Hypertension, medionecrosis (as in Marfan's syndrome). Most, however, are secondary to atheromatous disease.

12.   Acute abdomen with shock and pulsatile swelling from rupture.

13.   'Divers' bends — decompression syndrome from bubbles of nitrogen in the blood.

14.   10 per cent.

15.   60—70 per cent.

16.   Examples are Raynaud's disease, hyperhydrosis, concomitant with arterial surgery or in an ischaemic limb not amenable to vascular surgery, causalgia.

17.   Supraclavicular, axillary, posterior approach through necks of thoracic ribs.

18.   Endarterectomy of diseased segment.

19.   Elderly male with colicky abdominal pain after meals, associated with weight loss.

20.   Common effects are limb overgrowth or hypertrophy, ischaemic ulcers, eventual cardiac failure. If intracerebral it may cause subarachnoid haemorrhage.

1.   *The following features may be found in a patient with acute ischaemia of the leg*:

(a)   Loss of sensation in the foot
(b)   Atrial fibrillation
(c)   ECG changes of ischaemic heart disease
(d)   Blanching on elevation of the leg
(e)   Strong femoral pulsation

2.   *Which of the following may predispose to aneurysm formation*:

(a)   Subacute bacterial endocarditis
(b)   Trauma
(c)   Marfan's syndrome

(d)   Meig's syndrome
(e)   Ergot poisoning

3.   *The following features are commonly associated with a leaking aortic aneurysm*:

(a)   Blood staining in the loins
(b)   Oliguria
(c)   Calcification on plain abdominal X-ray
(d)   Blood-stained urine
(e)   Defibrination

4.   *The following conditions may give rise to Raynaud's syndrome*:

(a)   Hereditary telangiectasia
(b)   Scleroderma
(c)   Coeliac disease
(d)   Systemic lupus erythematosus
(e)   Macroglobulinaemia

5.   *In chronic arterial occlusion of the lower limbs*:

(a)   Elevation of the leg frequently relieves rest pain
(b)   The most commonly occluded major vessel is the superficial femoral artery
(c)   Buttock claudication occurs in aorto-iliac disease
(d)   Associated peripheral neuropathy is usual
(e)   Gangrene usually commences in the heel skin

Target scores U.G. 11, P.G. 17

1. (a) T   Loss of sensation to touch and prick is early in acute ischaemia
   (b) T ⎫ Atrial fibrillation and myocardial infarction are the commonest
   (c) T ⎭ causes of arterial emboli
   (d) T   Blanching on elevation occurs if the distal pressure falls significantly
   (e) T   An exaggerated femoral pulse often occurs proximal to an acute block

2. (a) T   Subacute bacterial endocarditis may give rise to mycotic aneurysms
   (b) T   Both false aneurysms or A–V fistula can occur
   (c) T   Medionecrosis leading to aortic dissection is more common in patients
            with Marfan's syndrome
   (d) F   This is serosal effusion secondary to an ovarian fibroma
   (e) F   This can produce acute ischaemia or Raynaud's phenomena

3. (a) F   This is uncommon
   (b) T   Due to hypotension or renal artery involvement
   (c) T   Many aneurysms calcify
   (d) F ⎫ These are rare
   (e) F ⎭

4. (a) F   This condition may produce gastro-intestinal haemorrhage
   (b) T
   (c) F
   (d) T   Most collagen diseases may develop Raynaud's phenomena
   (e) T   Possibly due to sludging of distal vessels

5. (a) F   Relief is obtained by hanging the leg down
   (b) T   This is the commonest site for atheroma in the leg
   (c) T   Aorto-iliac block produces the Leriche syndrome
   (d) F   Only in diabetics
   (e) F   Gangrene usually commences in the toes, although pressure necrosis
            in the heel may occur

25 VASCULAR SURGERY
   — VEINS AND LYMPHATICS

1.　　　　Name three methods of treatment for varicose veins.　　　　(1)

2.　　　　Name two complications of varicose veins.　　　　(1)

3.　　　　Name two common sites for perforating veins in the lower limb.　　　　(1)

4.　　　　What clinical features differentiate a saphena varix from a femoral hernia?　　　　(1)

5.　　　　What is the principle of sclerotherapy for varicose veins?　　　　(2)

6.　　　　Name two investigations to detect deep vein thrombosis.　　　　(2)

7.　　　　Name one effective method for prophylaxis of thrombo-embolism.　　　　(2)

8.　　　　Name three factors that increase the risk of thrombo-embolism.　　　　(2)

9.　　　　Name five causes of enlarged lymph nodes.　　　　(2)

10.　　　　Name three causes of lymphoedema.　　　　(2)

11.　　　　What is a Trendelenburg operation?　　　　(2)

12.　　　　Name two causes of secondary varicose veins of the leg.　　　　(2)

13.　　　　How do you diagnose a pulmonary embolus?　　　　(2)

14.　　　　What is the management of recurrent pulmonary emboli?　　　　(3)

15.　　　　What is the cause of phlegmasia caerulea dolens?　　　　(3)

16.　　　　Give three differential diagnoses for venous ulcer of the leg.　　　　(3)

17.　　　　What is a cystic hygroma?　　　　(3)

18.　　　　What is the commonest site for a lymphangioma?　　　　(3)

19.　　　　What is the operation usually required following treatment of a venous ulcer?　　　　(3)

20.　　　　What is Milroy's disease?　　　　(3)

Target scores U.G. 20, P.G. 30, max. 43

25 VASCULAR SURGERY
— VEINS AND LYMPHATICS

1. Sclerotherapy, surgery, elastic stockings.

2. Varicose eczema, venous ulcer, bleeding from traumatised varix, superficial thrombophlebitis, occasionally oedema or DVT.

3. Saphenofemoral junction (over Hunter's canal), pretibial perforators (near ankle).

4. Saphenavarix disappears on lying down; fluid thrill on coughing and tapping saphenous vein.

5. The sclerosing fluid produces localised acute phlebitis near the junction of a perforating vein. Compression then helps adherence of opposing walls of the vein, hindering recanalisation.

6. ^{131}I-labelled fibrogen scan, phlebography. Doppler ultrasound, impedance plethysmography.

7. Subcutaneous heparin, anticoagulation, calf muscle stimulation or intermittent compression, early mobilisation, graded compression stockings.

8. Age, immobility, major abdominal and pelvic surgery, splenectomy, polycythaemia, obesity, malignant disease, pregnancy and contraceptive pill.

9. Examples are acute or chronic lymphadenitis, either non-specific or specific (for example TB, syphilis); primary neoplasms such as Hodgkin's disease; secondary carcinoma, or part of a generalised lymphadenopathy, for example glandular fever, leukaemia, brucellosis.

10. Congenital hypoplasia or absence of lymphatics, chronic lymphadenitis, blocked drainage of regional lymph nodes (for example breast carcinoma), radiotherapy to regional lymph nodes, elephantiasis.

11. Ligation of the saphenofemoral junction and its tributaries.

12. Pregnancy, pelvic masses and previous iliac vein thrombosis.

13. Post-operative acute chest pain, pleural rub, haemoptysis, collapse, acute right-heart failure, confirmation by ECG, chest X-ray, pulmonary scan, possibly pulmonary angiography, demonstration of deep-vein thrombosis.

14. Bilateral leg phlebography to demonstrate origin. Streptokinase, thrombectomy or caval umbrella or ligation.

15. Iliofemoral thrombosis.

16. Ischaemic ulcer, malignant ulcer, ulcers complicating acholuric jaundice, ulcerative colitis, diabetic ulcers, traumatic ulcers, arteriovenous fistulas, chronic inflammatory ulcers (for example, syphilitic and tropical ulcers) or underlying osteomyelitis.

17. Congenital lymph cyst usually in the neck.

18. The tongue.

19. Subfascial ligation of perforators above the ankle.

20. Familial congenital lymphoedema.

1.   *The following statements are true of venous ulcers of the lower limbs*:

(a)   Classically they affect the lateral side of the leg
(b)   Most ulcers can be healed with dressings and pressure bandages
(c)   Bleeding can be stopped by elevating the leg
(d)   The ulcer may rarely turn malignant
(e)   Systemic antibiotics are required for most venous ulcers

2.   *Varicose veins of the lower limb*:

(a)   Are more common in the left leg
(b)   Most commonly occur in the short saphenous system
(c)   Are usually due to incompetent perforating veins
(d)   Are usually due to the iliac compression syndrome
(e)   Are more common in females

3.   *In the treatment of varicose veins*:

(a)   A Trendelenburg operation implies stripping of the long saphenous vein

(b)   Injection of phenol in almond oil is the usual method of sclerotherapy
(c)   Removal of all the superficial veins in the leg is commonly performed
(d)   Compression pads and bandaging for 4—6 weeks improves the results of injection therapy
(e)   One week of bed rest after surgery should be routine

4.   *In the prophylaxis of thrombo-embolism after surgery the following are effective*:

(a)   Intermittent calf compression at surgery
(b)   Oral heparin
(c)   Prostaglandin E systemically
(d)   High fluid intake to reduce viscosity
(e)   Post-operative calf massage

5.   *The following may cause chronic lymphoedema*:

(a)   Congenital lymphatic hypoplasia
(b)   Filariasis
(c)   Radical mastectomy
(d)   Chronic lymphadenitis
(e)   Radiotherapy

Target scores U.G. 16, P.G. 21

1. (a) F   Medial side is much commoner
   (b) T   Few ulcers will not respond to cleaning and adequate bandaging
   (c) T   Bleeding from an ulcer or varicose vein can be stopped by elevation
   (d) T   The so-called Marjolin's ulcer
   (e) F   Local antiseptics are usually adequate to control infection

2. (a) T   Possibly related to the crossing of the left common iliac artery
   (b) F   Less than 1 in 10 patients have short saphenous incompetence
   (c) T   Failure of the valves in perforating veins are the basic problem
   (d) F   This is rarely a true cause of venous incompetence
   (e) T

3. (a) F   A Trendelenburg operation is ligation of the saphenofemoral junction and its tributaries
   (b) F   This is the injection for piles!
   (c) F   This would be impossible!
   (d) T   Fegan's technique of sclerotherapy. The pads help sclerosis and prevent recanalisation
   (e) F   Early mobilisation is safer

4. (a) T
   (b) F   Heparin is ineffective given orally
   (c) F ⎫
   (d) F ⎬ There is no evidence of benefit of these measures
   (e) F ⎭

5. (a) T   As in Milroy's disease
   (b) T   This is a common cause of 'elephantiasis' in the tropics
   (c) T   Especially if followed by radiotherapy
   (d) T   Severe chronic infection can block lymphatic outflow
   (e) T

1.   Name four electrolyte solutions useful for intravenous infusion.   (1)

2.   What is the most commonly used replacement fluid in cases of severe burns?   (1)

3.   What would be your intravenous fluid of choice in intestinal obstruction?   (1)

4.   What would be your intravenous fluid of choice in a cardiac arrest?   (1)

5.   Why should blood be taken for cross-matching before giving intravenous dextran?   (1)

6.   What are the symptoms of acute hypocalcaemia?   (1)

7.   Name a common cause of respiratory acidosis.   (1)

8.   Name a cause of respiratory alkalosis.   (2)

9.   Name a cause for metabolic acidosis.   (2)

10.   Name a cause for metabolic alkalosis.   (2)

11.   What volume of fluid does the average patient require per 24 hours in a post-operative infusion?   (2)

12.   What are the physical symptoms and signs of potassium deficiency?   (3)

13.   What are the ECG signs of potassium depletion?   (3)

14.   What is the normal potassium concentration of the extracellular fluid?   (3)

15.   Name two causes of hypercalcaemia.   (3)

16.   What is the normal daily requirement of sodium?   (3)

17.   What is the normal daily requirement of potassium?   (3)

18.   What are the symptoms of water intoxication?   (3)

19.   What is the emergency treatment for hyperkalaemia?   (3)

20.   Name a cause of hypomagnesaemia.   (3)

Target scores U.G. 17, P.G. 26, max. 42

1.   The most commonly used solutions are normal saline 0.9 per cent, dextrose 5 per cent, dextrose-saline, Hartmann's solution, sodium lactate, sodium bicarbonate.

2.   Plasma or possibly plasma substitute — the solution must contain colloid. Severe burns will also require blood.

3.   Normal saline with added potassium; or Hartmann's solution.

4.   Sodium bicarbonate (there is a severe metabolic acidosis).

5.   Dextran interferes with cross-matching because of rouleaux formation.

6.   Paraesthesia in the limbs. Carpopedal spasm and tetany.

7.   Atelectasis and chest infection, especially in a patient with chronic bronchitis and emphysema.

8.   Over-breathing (for example in hysteria), severe peritonitis, salicylate poisoning.

9.   Increased production of acids by tissues — diabetic ketoacidosis; failure to remove or excrete acid — cardiac arrest, shock, renal failure; increased loss of base — diarrhoea.

10.   Ingestion of alkali; loss of acid (for example prolonged vomiting); excess urinary acid excretion (Conn's syndrome, Cushing's syndrome, for example).

11.   2–2½ litres.

12.   Muscle weakness, lethargy, paralytic ileus.

13.   Flat or absent T-waves ('No pot, no T').

14.   3.5–5 mmol/litre.

15.   Hyperparathyroidism, multiple bony metastases, vitamin D intoxication, sarcoidosis. Multiple myeloma milk-alkali syndrome.

16.   Adult: 80–120 mmol per 24 hours.

17.   80–100 mmol per 24 hours in adults.

18.   Headache, nausea, vomiting, abdominal cramps, weakness, stupor, coma and convulsions.

19.   Intravenous glucose with insulin, sodium bicarbonate and calcium. Less severe cases — ion exchange resin, potassium-depleting diuretics such as Lasix; with renal failure haemodialysis will be necessary.

20.   Chronic alcoholism, severe starvation, diarrhoea, malabsorption, hypo-parathyroidism, vitamin D intoxication.

1.   *The following are normal values for an adult male*:

(a)   Body water 60 per cent of total body weight
(b)   Blood pH 8.15
(c)   Insensible fluid loss is about 200 ml per 24 hours in temperate climates
(d)   Serum sodium 3.9—5.0 mmol/litre

(e)   Plasma volume 4 litres

2.   *A patient is admitted with high jejunal obstruction. The following features are likely to be found*:

(a)   Metabolic acidosis
(b)   Hyponatraemia
(c)   Hyperchloraemic acidosis
(d)   Reduced skin tension
(e)   Hyperkalaemia

3.   *In a patient with severe hypokalaemia the following may be found*:

(a)   Severe restlessness
(b)   Carpopedal spasm
(c)   Brisk knee jerks
(d)   Positive Trousseau's sign
(e)   Paralytic ileus

4.   *A patient presents with a serum potassium of 7.6 mmol/litre; the following may be indicated*:

(a)   Exchange transfusion
(b)   Haemodialysis
(c)   Intravenous calcium phosphate
(d)   Intravenous glucose/insulin
(e)   Oral ion-exchange resin

5.   *The following conditions may give rise to hypercalcaemia*:

(a)   Bone metastases from breast cancer
(b)   Buerger's disease
(c)   Vitamin D excess
(d)   Hysterical over-breathing
(e)   Sarcoidosis

Target scores U.G. 11, P.G. 17

1. (a) T   A 70 kg male contains some 42 litres of water
   (b) F   Normal pH is kept very close to 7.4
   (c) F   Loss from skin and lungs is nearer 1000 ml
   (d) F   These are the normal values for potassium (sodium = 135–145 mmol/litre)
   (e) T   Less for a woman

2. (a) F   Alkalosis would be likely from vomiting
   (b) T   Very common
   (c) F
   (d) T   Due to clinical dehydration and sodium loss
   (e) F   Potassium would also be lost with vomiting, although a low potassium may be masked by alkalosis

3. (a) F   Lethargy and weakness are commoner
   (b) F   This occurs in hypocalcaemia and severe alkalosis
   (c) F   Reduced jerks may occur
   (d) F   See (b)
   (e) T   Ileus is common in hypokalaemia

4. (a) F   This is unnecessary
   (b) T   This may be required if cause is acute renal failure
   (c) F   Calcium would not help hyperkalaemia
   (d) T   Glucose/insulin is used in emergency treatment of hyperkalaemia
   (e) T   Ion-exchange resin (for example Resonium A) will help remove potassium from the body

5. (a) T   Hypercalcaemia is not uncommon with bone metastases
   (b) F
   (c) T   Vitamin D increases calcium absorption
   (d) F
   (e) T   Sarcoidosis can lead to hypercalcaemia

1.   Name three types of shock.   (1)

2.   Name four clinical features in shock.   (1)

3.   What is the commonest cause of hypovolaemic shock?   (1)

4.   Name three causes of hypovolaemic shock.   (1)

5.   How do you diagnose vasovagal neurogenic shock?   (1)

6.   For how long can the brain stand circulatory arrest before cell death occurs at normal body temperature?   (1)

7.   What is the significance of the urinary output in shock?   (2)

8.   What is the significance of a high central venous pressure?   (2)

9.   What is the normal range of central venous pressure measured from right atrial level?   (2)

10.   What are the two priorities in the treatment of hypovolaemic shock? (2)

11.   What is the commonest organism to produce Gram-negative shock? (2)

12.   What is the effect of severe prolonged shock on the kidney?   (2)

13.   How may the central venous pressure distinguish myocardial infarction and pulmonary embolism from hypovolaemic shock? (2)

14.   Name two drugs that may improve tissue perfusion in severe septic shock.   (3)

15.   Name two antibiotics useful in Gram-negative septicaemia.   (3)

16.   Name two common operations not infrequently complicated by Gram-negative septicaemia.   (3)

17.   What drugs are commonly used in the treatment of anaphylactic shock?(3)

18.   What would be an indication for giving heparin to a patient with shock?(3)

19.   What is principally responsible for pulmonary insufficiency in severe shock?   (3)

20.   Name two causes of shock, associated with a high CVP.   (3)

Target scores U.G. 17, P.G. 26, max. 41

1.   Common types are neurogenic shock, hypovolaemic shock, septic shock, cardiogenic shock and anaphylactic shock.

2.   Dizziness, faintness, sweating, tachycardia, hypotension, pallor.

3.   Bleeding.

4.   External haemorrhage, haematemesis and melaena, severe burns, severe fluid and electrolyte deficiency (for example gross intestinal obstruction).

5.   It is usually precipitated by emotional cause and rapidly recovers when the patient lies flat.

6.   Classically four minutes, but in practice variable.

7.   Urinary output is the best guide to tissue perfusion of vital organs.

8.   High central venous pressure indicates pump failure (for example cardiac failure, cardiac tamponade, pulmonary embolism and fluid overload).

9.   Plus 5—15 cm of water.

10.   Rapid replacement of blood volume, maintenance of adequate airway, adequate perfusion of vital organs, and of course stopping the bleeding!

11.   Coliform organisms.

12.   Acute tubular necrosis or acute corticol necrosis.

13.   In myocardial infarction and pulmonary embolism the central venous pressure is high. In hypovolaemic shock it is low.

14.   Isoprenalin, phenoxybenzamine, high doses of steroids, dopamine.

15.   Drugs of value are gentamycin, carbenicillin, cephalosporins, colistin, clindamycin, tobramycin, amikacin.

16.   Operations on the urinary tract with infected urine (for example prostatectomy), cholecystectomy with infected bile, and large-bowel resection.

17.   Parenteral adrenaline, antihistamines, steroids.

18.   Disseminated intravascular coagulation, pulmonary embolism.

19.   Pulmonary microembolism.

20.   Myocardial infarction, acute heart failure, pulmonary embolism.

1. *The following clinical features are common in a shocked patient*:

(a) Peripheral cyanosis
(b) Sweating
(c) Purpura
(d) Thirst
(e) Cheyne—Stokes breathing

2. *The following conditions may give rise to acute hypovolaemic shock*:

(a) Pulmonary embolism
(b) Acute right heart failure
(c) High jejunal obstruction
(d) Dumping syndrome
(e) Pancreatitis

3. *The following types of operation may precipitate Gram-negative septicaemia*:

(a) Transurethral resection

(b) Cholecystectomy
(c) Millin's prostatectomy
(d) Drainage of a quinsy
(e) Myringotomy

4. *A rising blood pressure and falling pulse rate are signs of*:

(a) Acute hypovolaemic shock
(b) Septicaemic shock
(c) Raised intracranial pressure
(d) Stokes—Adam's attack
(e) Carcinoid syndrome

5. *Which of the following drugs may be useful in shock*:

(a) Ouabaine
(b) Adrenaline
(c) Carbenicillin
(d) Phthalylsulphathiazole
(e) Phenoxybenzamine

Target scores U.G. 14, P.G. 19

1. (a) T In shock there is often marked peripheral arteriolar vasoconstriction
   (b) T
   (c) F
   (d) T
   (e) F

2. (a) F ⎫ Shock is not due to hypovolaemia
   (b) F ⎭
   (c) T Severe electrolyte and fluid loss can cause hypovolaemic shock
   (d) F This syndrome does not give rise to shock
   (e) T Hypovolaemia is common in acute pancreatitis

3. (a) T Any urinary tract procedure in the presence of urinary infection is at
            risk
   (b) T Gram-negative organisms frequently infect the biliary tree
   (c) T As for (a)
   (d) F *Staphylococcus aureus* is commonly the cause of a peritonsillar abscess
   (e) F This is incision of the eardrum for a severe otitis media

4. (a) F ⎫ The opposite would occur in shock
   (b) F ⎭
   (c) T This is the characteristic sign of progressive raised intracranial pressure
   (d) F
   (e) F

5. (a) T This drug has rapid digitalis-like effects
   (b) T In anaphylactic shock
   (c) T Useful in pseudomonas septicaemia
   (d) F No value in shock — useful in bowel preparation
   (e) T This drug may be indicated in severe septic shock not responding to
            fluids and antibiotics

1.   What is a paronychia?   (1)

2.   What is the commonest cystic lesion of the hand and wrist?   (1)

3.   Which nerve supplies most of the skin of the hand?   (1)

4.   Which nerve supplies most of the intrinsic muscles of the hand?   (1)

5.   What is a trigger finger?   (1)

6.   What are the features of carpal tunnel syndrome?   (2)

7.   What is the treatment of carpal tunnel syndrome?   (2)

8.   What is the surgical treatment of Dupuytren's contracture?   (2)

9.   Name two conditions associated with Dupuytren's contracture.   (2)

10.   What is the cause of a 'buttonhole' deformity?   (2)

11.   What is the cause of mallet finger?   (2)

12.   What is the treatment of mallet finger?   (2)

13.   What is a Bennett's fracture?   (2)

14.   What are the physical signs of tenosynovitis?   (2)

15.   Name two hand operations that may be indicated in rheumatoid
arthritis.   (3)

16.   What is the commonest malignancy in the hand?   (3)

17.   What is the commonest bone tumour of the hand?   (3)

18.   What is the commonest congenital anomaly of the hand?   (3)

19.   What is a felon?   (3)

20.   What are the clinical features of *Herpes simplex* infection of the
finger?   (3)

Target scores U.G. 18, P.G. 28, max. 41

1.   An infection of the nail fold.

2.   A ganglion.

3.   Median nerve,

4.   Ulnar nerve.

5.   Stenosing flexor tenovaginitis (bulge in tendon wedges in flexion and suddenly releases with a snap).

6.   Aching forearm and hand, associated paraesthesia, later wasting in distribution of median nerve. Symptoms are worse at night and occur usually in middle-aged females.

7.   Steroid injection may help early cases but most require division of carpal tunnel roof (the flexor retinaculum). Any underlying cause, such as myxoedema, should be treated.

8.   Fasciectomy.

9.   Cirrhosis, epilepsy, supraclavicular fat pads, Dupuytren's contracture of the foot, Peyronie's disease.

10.   Hyperextension of the distal phalangeal joint and flexion of the proximal intraphalangeal joint due to attenuation or rupture of the central part of the extensor tendon where it is inserted into the middle phalanx.

11.   Mallet finger is due to stretching or rupture of the extensor insertion into the distal phalanx producing acute flexion deformity of the terminal interphalangeal joint.

12.   Splinting in full extension for six weeks.

13.   Unstable fracture dislocation of the base of the 1st metacarpal in the thumb.

14.   Local tenderness and pain on active or passive stretching of the tendons. There may be some associated crepitus.

15.   Conditions amenable to surgery include synovectomy for boggy synovitis of tendons and joints, correction of tendon rupture, release of stenosing tenosynovitis and median and ulnar nerve compressions, excision of rheumatoid nodules, replacement of metacarpophalangeal and proximal phalangeal joints.

16.   Squamous cell carcinoma of the dorsum of the hand.

17.   Enchondroma.

18.   Syndactyly.

19.   Infection of the distal fat pad of the finger.

20.   Severe pain, multiple tiny vesicles particularly of the distal phalanx.

1.   *Sepsis of the hand commonly manifests as*:

(a)   Suppurative tenosynovitis
(b)   Nail fold infection
(c)   Web space infection
(d)   Pulp space infection
(e)   *Herpes* arthritis

2. *   *Flexor tendon injuries*:

(a)   Need immediate tendon grafting
(b)   In the fingers usually respond to immediate suturing
(c)   Often require secondary repair
(d)   At the wrist should have immediate suture
(e)   Have a better prognosis than extensor injuries

3.   *Carpal tunnel syndrome can be caused by*:

(a)   Fracture at the wrist
(b)   Cervical rib
(c)   Rheumatoid arthritis
(d)   Myxoedema
(e)   Syringomyelia

4.   *Carpal tunnel syndrome includes*:

(a)   Wasting of the hypothenar muscles
(b)   Discomfort in the arm and hand at night
(c)   Weakness of the first dorsal interosseus muscle
(d)   Loss of sensation in the little finger
(e)   Blanching of the skin with cold exposure

5.   *Radial nerve injury may produce*:

(a)   Main-en-griffe
(b)   Thenar eminence paralysis
(c)   Paralysis of flexor carpi ulnaris
(d)   Wrist drop
(e)   A small patch of anaesthesia only

Target scores U.G. 13, P.G. 19

1. (a)   Γ   Septic tendon sheath infection is rare
   (b)   T   This is a paronychia
   (c)   T   Infection between the fingers is not uncommon
   (d)   T   Finger-tip pulp infection from pricks and cuts
   (e)   F

2. (a)   F ⎫   Flexor tendon injuries within the sheaths do not respond well to
   (b)   F ⎬   primary repair. Wound closure and delayed grafting or suture is
   (c)   T ⎭   routine
   (d)   T   At the wrist, adhesion to flexor sheaths is not a problem
   (e)   F   Functional result is worse

3. (a)   T   Any cause of compression of the carpal tunnel can cause the syndrome
   (b)   F   This can cause the 'thoracic outlet syndrome' and Raynaud's attacks
   (c)   T ⎫
            ⎬ See (a)
   (d)   T ⎭
   (e)   F

4. (a)   F   Thenar muscles
   (b)   T   Symptoms are often worst at night
   (c)   F   Nearly always supplied by the ulnar nerve
   (d)   F   This would be ulnar nerve
   (e)   F   No colour change occurs

5. (a)   F   This is ulnar nerve damage
   (b)   F
   (c)   F
   (d)   T   The radial nerve supplies extensors of the wrist
   (e)   T   Due to overlap, the sensory loss is usually a small patch over the first
            dorsal interosseus muscle area

1. Name four types of arthritis. (1)

2. What is the commonest organism to produce osteomyelitis? (1)
3. What is the commonest operation for osteo-arthritis of the hip? (1)
4. Name four causes of low back pain. (1)

5. Name three clinical features of a prolapsed lumbar intervertebral disc. (1)

6. Which are the commonest joints to be involved in rheumatoid arthritis? (1)
7. What is the commonest type of clubfoot? (1)
8. What is the common age group and site for osteosarcoma? (2)
9. What is Charcot's disease? (2)
10. What is Perthe's disease? (2)

11. Name two causes of paraplegia. (2)

12. What is the cause of, and an alternative name for, osteitis fibrosa cystica? (2)
13. Name three primary bone tumours. (3)

14. Give the sex incidence and clinical features of ankylosing spondylitis? (3)

15. What is spondylolisthesis? (3)

16. Name three causes of the 'painful arc' syndrome. (3)

17. What are the two commonest sites of Paget's disease of bone? (3)
18. Name three causes of locking of the knee. (3)

19. What is the nail—patella syndrome? (3)
20. In what condition do you find Looser's zones on an X-ray? (3)

Target scores U.G. 18, P.G. 27, max. 41

1.   Types include osteo-arthritis, rheumatoid arthritis, acute suppurative arthritis, gonococcal arthritis, tuberculous arthritis, gouty arthritis.

2.   *Staphylococcus pyogenes.*

3.   Now, total hip replacement.

4.   Numerous causes include (1) injury, such as muscle injury, prolapsed disc, compression fracture; (2) degeneration, such as scoliosis, kyphosis, lumbar spondylosis; (3) spinal disease, such as ankylosing spondylitis, secondary deposits, Paget's disease; (4) referred pain, from, for example, aneurysm, carcinoma of the ovary, carcinoma of the rectum, carcinoma of the cervix, retroperitoneal fibrosis; (5) idiopathic, such as sacro-iliac strain.

5.   Clinical features include sudden onset of severe back pain on lifting or stooping, frequently associated with sciatica, pain made worse by coughing or straining; there may be associated paraesthesia. Examination shows spasm and scoliosis, limitation of straight-leg raising and back movements. There may be reduced sensation in the leg, and muscle weakness, most commonly in the distribution of L5 or S1. Ankle jerk may be diminished.

6.   The wrist, fingers and toes — especially interphalangeal and metacarpophalangeal joints.

7.   Talipes equinovarus.

8.   Children; metaphysis of long bone frequently near the knee.

9.   A neuropathic joint, classically caused by syphilis.

10.   A condition in which the femoral head becomes partly or wholly avascular; occurs in children.

11.   Causes include trauma to the spine, compression from secondary deposits in the spine, spinal cord tumours, disseminated sclerosis and spina bifida, infections such as tuberculosis, poliomyelitis.

12.   Von Recklinghausen's disease of bone caused by primary hyperparathyroidism.

13.   Numerous tumours include osteoma, osteosarcoma, chondroma, Ewing's tumour, myeloma, haemangioma, fibrosarcoma, osteoclastoma.

14.   Much commoner in men, age group 15 — 35, presents with pain and stiffness in the lumbar spine and buttocks. 25 per cent have associated iritis, 10 per cent have polyarthritis. Examination shows stiffness of the lumbar spine.

15.   Forward shift of the spine, nearly always between L4 and L5; may be congenital due to defective superior sacral facets, degenerative or spondylolitic, rarely traumatic.

16.   Causes include supraspinatus tear, acute supraspinatus tendinitis, supraspinatus tendon calcification, subachromial bursitis, fracture of greater tuberosity of the humerus.

17.   The pelvis and the tibia.

18.   Torn meniscus, loose body e.g. osteochondritis dissecans, after haemarthrosis or synovitis or neuropathic arthritis, recurrent dislocation of the patella.

19.   Familial hypoplasia of the nails and patella.

20.   Osteomalacia.

1.   *Acute osteomyelitis*:

(a)   Is more common in Paget's disease
(b)   Is usually caused by *Streptococcus pyogenes*
(c)   Often starts in the metaphysis
(d)   Is commoner in children
(e)   Usually requires bone drilling

2.   *Osteosarcoma*:

(a)   Is the commonest primary tumour of bone
(b)   Is usually a spindle cell tumour
(c)   Usually involves a long bone
(d)   Spreads early to lymph nodes
(e)   Always requires amputation

3.   *A torn cartilage in the knee*:

(a)   Commonly presents in the elderly
(b)   Usually involves the lateral cartilage
(c)   Frequently produces locking in extension
(d)   Often leads to crepitus of the patellofemoral joint
(e)   Leads to a positive McBurney's test

4.   *A prolapsed lumbar disc*:

(a)   Usually affects L4—5 or L5—S1 discs
(b)   May cause loss of ankle reflex
(c)   Often leads to pain worse on sneezing and coughing
(d)   Requires routine myelography

(e)   Usually requires laminectomy

5.   *Gout*:

(a)   Most commonly affects the hips and knees
(b)   May affect the kidneys
(c)   Usually starts in the third decade
(d)   Rarely deforms joints
(e)   Is often associated with hypercalciuria

Target scores U.G. 13, P.G. 18

1. (a)   F   Although osteosarcoma is
   (b)   F   Most cases are still due to *Staphylococcus aureus*
   (c)   T
   (d)   T
   (e)   F   Most early cases respond to adequate antibiotic therapy

2. (a)   T
   (b)   F   Anaplastic pleomorphic cells are usual
   (c)   T   Most cases occur in limb long bones
   (d)   F   Blood spread is usual
   (e)   F   Primary treatment is radiotherapy, and amputation considered if no metastases are apparent after course of treatment

3. (a)   F   It is a disease of active young adults
   (b)   F   Medial cartilage is commoner
   (c)   F   The limb locks in a flexed position
   (d)   F
   (e)   F   McBurney talked about the appendix — try McMurray!

4. (a)   T   These are the commonest to be affected
   (b)   T
   (c)   T
   (d)   F   Myelography is indicated only if laminectomy is considered, or diagnosis is in doubt
   (e)   F   Most cases can be treated conservatively

5. (a)   F   Small joints are usually affected
   (b)   T   Nephropathy is not rare
   (c)   F   Gout is commoner in the elderly
   (d)   F   Deformity of small joints affected is common
   (e)   F   Excess uric acid excretion is common and may give rise to uric acid calculi

1.   What is a greenstick fracture?   (1)

2.   What is the commonest cause of a fractured clavicle?   (1)

3.   Name three complications of fractures.   (1)

4.   Give three causes of a pathological fracture.   (1)

5.   What is malunion?   (1)

6.   What is the commonest site for a fractured femur?   (1)

7.   What is the commonest fracture over the age of 40?   (1)

8.   Name three common fractures caused by a fall on the outstretched
hand.   (2)

9.   What is the common cause of a compression fracture of the calcaneum? (2)

10.   What is a 'march' fracture?   (2)

11.   Name two common sites of spinal fractures.   (2)

12.   What are three causes of non-union of a fracture?   (3)

13.   Name two fractures liable to result in vascular injury.   (3)

14.   Name two common sites of avascular necrosis.   (3)

15.   What are the common presenting features of fat embolism?   (3)

16.   Name an operation for recurrent dislocation of the shoulder.   (3)

17.   What is a Smith's fracture?   (3)

18.   What are three types of fracture-dislocation of the hip?   (3)

19.   What is a 'bumper' fracture?   (3)

20.   What is a Monteggia fracture—dislocation?   (3)

Target scores U.G. 18, P.G. 27, max. 42

1.   Fractures characteristically seen in children where the bone ends remain partly in continuity.

2.   A fall on the outstretched hand.

3.   Complications include infection if compound, injury of surrounding structures (for example arteries and nerves), malunion, delayed union, non-union, fat embolism.

4.   Many causes include secondary tumours, primary bone tumours, fibrous dysplasia, bone cyst, osteoporosis, hyperparathyroidism, Paget's disease.

5.   Malunion is when the fracture unites in a deformed position.

6.   The neck of the femur.

7.   Colles' fracture of the wrist.

8.   Common fractures include Colles' fracture, fractured clavicle, fractured scaphoid, fractured head or neck of radius.

9.   Fall onto the heel from a height.

10.   Stress fracture of the metatarsals — usually second.

11.   Cervical spine and lumbar spine.

12.   Failure of adequate splintage, wide separation of fracture ends, interposition of soft tissues, unrecognised pathological fracture, avascular necrosis, infection.

13.   Supracondylar fracture of the humerus, fractures of the lower end of the femur, rarely dislocation of shoulder, fracture of humerus and femoral shaft.

14.   Common sites are the head of the femur, scaphoid and lunate; less commonly talus, head of humerus.

15.   Dyspnoea due to pulmonary oedema; brain causing restlessness, drowsiness, vomiting; skin producing a purpuric rash particularly on the chest.

16.   Bankart or Putti—Platt.

17.   Fracture—dislocation of the lower end of the radius with anterior displacement of the distant fragment.

18.   Anterior, posterior and central.

19.   Fracture of the lateral condyle of the tibia, classically caused by a car bumper.

20.   Fracture of the upper end of the ulnar with dislocation of the head of the radius.

1.   *In a Colles' fracture the displacements of the distal fragments include*:

(a)   Rotation posteriorly
(b)   Ulnar deviation
(c)   Supination
(d)   Impaction to the radial side
(e)   Pronation

2.   *In a patient with dislocation of the shoulder*:

(a)   The head of humerus is frequently subcoracoid
(b)   Posterior dislocation is usual
(c)   The deltoid muscle may be paralysed
(d)   The dislocation can be reduced by Bilroth's manoeuvre
(e)   Injury to the axillary artery rarely occurs

3.   *Which of the following fractures are commonly not detected on an early X-ray*:

(a)   Fractured styloid process
(b)   Fracture of carpal scaphoid
(c)   March fracture of metatarsal
(d)   Fractured greater tuberosity of humerus
(e)   Fracture of clavicle

4.   *Which of the following fractures may be complicated by avascular necrosis*:

(a)   Subcapital fracture of femoral neck
(b)   Fracture of lunate
(c)   Fracture of talus
(d)   Bennet's fracture of first metacarpal
(e)   Fracture of calcaneum

5.   *Which of the following fractures often require operative fixation*:

(a)   Fracture of ilium
(b)   Fracture of neck of femur
(c)   Fracture of neck of humerus
(d)   Scaphoid fracture
(e)   Fractured shaft of tibia

Target scores U.G. 11, P.G. 16

1. (a)   T ⎫
   (b)   F ⎪ In a Colles' fracture, radial fragment is displaced and impacted to the
   (c)   T ⎬   radial side, rotated posteriorly and supinated
   (d)   T ⎪
   (e)   F ⎭

2. (a)   T ⎫ Anterior displacement is commonest
   (b)   F ⎭
   (c)   T   Due to circumflex nerve injury
   (d)   F   Try Kocher's or Hippocrate's!
   (e)   T   Only occasionally in the elderly with an atherosclerotic vessel

3. (a)   F
   (b)   T ⎫ Both are often undisplaced hairline cracks
   (c)   T ⎭
   (d)   F
   (e)   F

4. (a)   T
   (b)   T   Blood supply crosses the neck into the head of the lunate
   (c)   T   Fortunately an uncommon fracture
   (d)   F
   (e)   F

5. (a)   F   Pelvic fractures rarely require surgery
   (b)   T   Either fixation or replacement of femoral head
   (c)   F
   (d)   F
   (e)   T   Most typical fractures are treated by open fixation

1.   What is the best nursing position for an unconscious patient following a head injury?   (1)

2.   What is the most important nursing observation following a head injury?   (1)

3.   What is the usual cause of an extradural haematoma?   (1)

4.   What changes may be seen in the pupils from an expanding intracranial haematoma?   (1)

5.   What is an internal compound fracture of the skull?   (2)

6.   What is the best guide to severity of concussion?   (2)

7.   Name two complications of a head injury not related to intracranial bleeding.   (2)

8.   What investigations may be helpful in localising intracranial haemorrhage?   (2)

9.   What causes dilatation of the pupil in an enlarging intracranial clot?   (2)

10.   How may one decide on which side to make burr holes in suspected extradural haematoma?   (2)

11.   Name four causes of coma other than head injuries.   (2)

12.   How can one distinguish CSF rhinorrhoea from nasal discharge?   (3)

13.   What is 'coning'?   (3)

14.   What are the accompanying physical signs that may be seen with an anterior fossa fracture?   (3)

15.   What are the accompanying physical signs that may be seen with a middle fossa fracture?   (3)

16.   How may one distinguish an orbital haematoma from a 'black-eye'?   (3)

17.   How do extradural and acute subdural haematoma differ clinically?   (3)

18.   What are the features of a chronic subdural haematoma?   (3)

19.   What is Kernig's sign?   (3)

20.   What is the management of CSF rhinorrhoea?   (3)

Target scores U.G. 18, P.G. 29, max. 45

1.   Semi-prone position with head turned to the side and lower than the body.

2.   Change in conscious level.

3.   A tear in the middle meningeal artery.

4.   Pupil on the side of an expanding haematoma dilates and fails to respond to light. As the compression continues the contralateral pupil also dilates and becomes fixed.

5.   Fracture involving a nasal sinus or the middle ear.

6.   The duration of pretraumatic amnesia.

7.   Brain damage, cervical spine damage, facial injuries, airway obstruction, meningitis, brain abscess, epilepsy.

8.   Ultrasound, angiography, EEG, brain scan, computerised axial tomography.

9.   Stretching of the 3rd cranial nerve over the edge of the tentorium cerebelli.

10.   The first set of burr holes should be made on the side of the skull fracture, the side of the dilated pupil, or the side in which ultrasound has suggested there is a haematoma. The CAT scan gives accurate localisation.

11.   Many causes include cerebrovascular accident, epilepsy, cerebral tumour, alcohol, carbon monoxide poisoning, barbiturate overdose, diabetic coma, uraemia, hepatic coma, meningitis.

12.   CSF discharge is increased by jugular compression, CSF contains sugar and no mucin, unlike nasal discharge.

13.   Compression of the brain stem as a result of raised intracranial pressure.

14.   Nasal bleeding, CSF rhinorrhoea, orbital haematoma, injuries to cranial nerves 1–6.

15.   Orbital haematoma, bleeding from the ear, injuries to cranial nerves 7 and 8.

16.   In an orbital haematoma there is no posterior limit to the haematoma; in a conjunctival haemorrhage a posterior limit is nearly always seen.

17.   In subdural haemorrhage there is usually a much severer head injury and coma from the moment of injury. In extradural haemorrhage there is frequently a lucid interval. There may, however, be no difference.

18.   Chronic subdural haematoma may follow a trivial injury, frequently of weeks or months before. Clinical features are those of a space-occupying lesion with headaches, vomiting, drowsiness and mental deterioration.

19.   Passive flexion of the hip to 90° causes spasm of the hamstrings such that it is impossible to straighten the knee.

20.   Most cases clear spontaneously, persistent cases require repair of the torn dura mater.

1. *Deterioration in a patient with head injury is determined by*:

(a) Serial EEGs
(b) Deepening conscious level
(c) Repeated angiography
(d) Pupil becoming fixed
(e) Computerised axial tomograms

2. *The following are relevant features of an anterior cranial fossa fracture*:

(a) Rhinorrhoea
(b) Anosmia
(c) Hyperacusis
(d) Facial palsy
(e) Orbital haematomas

3. *The features of a fracture of the zygoma may include*:

(a) Diplopia
(b) Supra-orbital anaesthesia
(c) Loss of taste
(d) Loss of sensation cheek
(e) Radio-opacity of the antrum

4. *Subdural haemorrhage*:

(a) Is usually due to bleeding from the middle meningeal artery
(b) A lucid interval is usual

(c) If chronic, may not have a history of head injury

(d) Has a worse prognosis than extradural haemorrhage
(e) Frequently requires an osteoplastic flap in management

5. *Indications for surgical intervention in head injuries are*:

(a) Epileptic fit
(b) Cerebral oedema
(c) Compound depressed fractures
(d) Fracture of petrous temporal bone
(e) Anosmia

Target scores U.G. 12, P.G. 18

1. (a)   F ⎫
     (b)   T ⎪
     (c)   F ⎬ Clinical observation is still the best guide to deterioration in head injuries
     (d)   T ⎪
     (e)   F ⎭

2. (a)   T   Cerebrospinal fluid leak is not uncommon if fracture involves sinuses
     (b)   T   First cranial nerve may be damaged
     (c)   F
     (d)   F
     (e)   T   Orbital haematomas are very common

3. (a)   T   If the floor of the orbit is displaced
     (b)   F   Infra-orbital nerve may be involved
     (c)   F
     (d)   T   See (b)
     (e)   T   Bleeding into the antrum may occur

4. (a)   F   This would be extradural — subdural is from cerebral veins
     (b)   F   This is much less common in acute subdural bleeding as the head injury is often more severe
     (c)   T   Chronic subdural haemorrhage occurs in the elderly, often with slight trauma
     (d)   T   From associated brain damage
     (e)   T   Burr holes are often inadequate to deal with the clot

5. (a)   F ⎫ Not unless associated with localising signs of a haematoma or
     (b)   F ⎭ deterioration in consciousness
     (c)   T   Compound depressed fractures require lifting
     (d)   F
     (e)   F

1.   What is spina bifida occulta?   (1)

2.   What is the treatment of progressive congenital hydrocephalus?   (1)

3.   What is the commonest presentation of an intracranial aneurysm?   (1)

4.   Name three special investigations in neurosurgery.   (1)

5.   What is the commonest primary brain tumour?   (1)

6.   What is the commonest cause of a brain abscess?   (1)

7.   Name three clinical features of increased intracranial pressure.   (1)

8.   Which brain tumour has the best prognosis?   (1)

9.   What is the commonest cause of non-traumatic subarachnoid
haemorrhage?   (2)

10.   Name three causes of an intracranial space-occupying lesion.   (2)

11.   What are the usual ocular manifestations of a pituitary tumour?   (2)

12.   Name three causes of a hydrocephalus.   (2)

13.   What are the clinical features of a radial nerve injury at the elbow? (2)

14.   What is the commonest tumour to cause spinal cord compression?   (3)

15.   Name three types of spinal cord tumour.   (3)

16.   What is a medulloblastoma?   (3)

17.   What is the commonest pituitary tumour?   (3)

18.   What are the features of a patient with eosinophil adenoma of the
pituitary?   (3)

19.   What produces the cerebellopontine angle syndrome?   (3)

20.   What is the Sturge—Weber syndrome?   (3)

Target scores U.G. 17, P.G. 27, max. 39

1.   Defect in the spinal arch without any neurological involvement.

2.   Insertion of a ventriculoatrial shunt, usually with a Spitz—Holter valve.

3.   Subarachnoid haemorrhage, occasionally epilepsy.

4.   Special investigations include ultrasound, brain scan, EEG, lumbar puncture, angiography, air encephalogram, ventriculography, computerised axial tomography (which has now replaced most of the latter).

5.   Glioma (commonest type astrocytoma).

6.   Middle ear infection.

7.   Headaches, nausea, vomiting, mental changes, papilloedema, vertigo, bradycardia, raised systolic blood pressure, pupillary dilatation.

8.   Meningioma.

9.   Ruptured berry aneurysm.

10.   Secondary tumours, primary brain tumours, cerebral abscess, chronic sub-dural haematoma.

11.   Bitemporal hemianopia.

12.   Causes include blockage within the duct system by tumour, abscess, congenital stenosis, failure of villus absorption due to meningitis, birth trauma.

13.   Wrist drop — paralysis of the extensors. There may be a small sensory loss over the dorsum of the hand near the thumb.

14.   Secondary deposits in the spine, commonly from bronchus, breast and prostate.

15.   Types include extradural (for example secondary deposits (commonest), multiple myeloma, reticuloses); intradural (meningioma, neurofibroma); intra-medullary (for example glioma, ependymoma).

16.   Rapidly growing tumour arising in the roof of the fourth ventricle in children, frequently presenting with obstructive hydrocephalus.

17.   Chromophobe adenoma.

18.   Gigantism or acromegaly.

19.   An acoustic nerve tumour.

20.   Congenital port-wine naevus of the face associated with cerebral angioma, usually on the opposite side of the brain.

1. *The following features are common in a cerebellar space-occupying lesion*:

(a) Fortification spectra
(b) Transient blackouts
(c) Ataxia
(d) Nystagmus
(e) Drooping eyelid

2. *The features of an acoustic neuroma may include*:

(a) Unilateral loss of taste
(b) Generalised neurofibromatosis
(c) Facial weakness
(d) Widening of the internal auditory meatus on X-ray
(e) Facial numbness

3. *A pituitary tumour may present with*:

(a) Bilateral central scotoma
(b) Hypothyroidism
(c) Hypoadrenalism
(d) Diabetes insipidus
(e) Thyrotoxicosis

4. *The following statements about intracranial aneurysms are correct*:

(a) Most are due to atherosclerosis
(b) Most are fusiform aneurysms
(c) Most occur on the anterior communicating arteries
(d) Most occur in men
(e) Most present with subdural haemorrhage

5. *A fracture–dislocation of T12–L1 will usually be followed by*:

(a) Permanent paralysis below T12 level in the cord
(b) Permanent hypotension from sympathetic damage
(c) Combined cord and cauda equina injury
(d) Exaggerated knee jerks
(e) Recovery of lumbar nerves

Target scores U.G. 10, P.G. 15

1. (a)   F   These occur in migraine or optic-track lesions
   (b)   F   These occur in vertebrobasilar attacks
   (c)   T } These are common in cerebellar lesions
   (d)   T }
   (e)   F   There would be no reason for a 3rd nerve palsy until severely raised intracranial pressure

2. (a)   T   From 7th nerve lesion
   (b)   T   Acoustic neuromas are commoner in Von Recklinghausen's disease
   (c)   T   7th nerve damage
   (d)   T   Common
   (e)   T   The lesion can involve the 5th cranial nerve (and 7th, 9th, 10th, 11th or 12th)

3. (a)   F   Bitemporal hemi-anopia
   (b)   T   From TSH deficiency
   (c)   T   Due to ACTH deficiency
   (d)   T   From lack of ADH
   (e)   F

4. (a)   F   Apart from micro-aneurysms, 95 per cent of aneurysms are congenital
   (b)   F   Saccular
   (c)   F   Middle cerebral and internal carotid account for 60 per cent
   (d)   F   Sex incidence is equal
   (e)   F   Subarachnoid haemorrhage

5. (a)   F }
   (b)   F } T12–L1 injury produces a cord lesion at S1 but lumbar nerve root
   (c)   T } involvement up to L1. The sacral paralysis will be permanent but the
   (d)   F } lumbar roots may recover with return of hip and knee movement
   (e)   T

1.	Name three methods of treating tumours.	(1)
2.	What is the difference between a sarcoma and a carcinoma?	(1)
3.	Name three sarcomas.	(1)
4.	Name two tumours highly sensitive to radiotherapy.	(1)
5.	Give two examples of hormone treatment of cancer.	(1)
6.	Name two complications of cancer chemotherapy.	(1)
7.	Give two examples of useful palliative treatment in cancer therapy.	(2)
8.	Give two examples of cancers with a very bad prognosis.	(2)
9.	Give two examples of cancers with a very good prognosis.	(2)
10.	Why is a carcinoid tumour so called?	(2)
11.	Give an example of immunotherapy.	(2)
12.	Name three chemotherapeutic agents for cancer treatment.	(2)
13.	Where would you find a cystosarcoma phylloides?	(3)
14.	Where would you find a glomus tumour?	(3)
15.	What is the commonest site for a liposarcoma?	(3)
16.	Name two malignant tumours of children.	(3)
17.	Where would you find an adenolymphoma?	(3)
18.	Where would you find a desmoid tumour?	(3)
19.	Where would you find a chemodectoma?	(3)
20.	What is Bowen's disease?	(3)

Target scores U.G. 18, P.G. 27, max. 42

1.　　Surgical excision, radiotherapy, chemotherapy, hormone therapy.

2.　　A sarcoma is a malignant tumour of connective tissue. Carcinoma is a malignant tumour of epithelial and glandular origin.

3.　　Examples are osteosarcoma, leiomyosarcoma, rhabdomyosarcoma, haemangiosarcoma, fibrosarcoma, chondrosarcoma.

4.　　Examples are neuroblastoma, Hodgkin's disease, seminoma of testis, reticulum cell sarcoma.

5.　　Androgen's for breast cancer, oestrogens for prostatic carcinoma.

6.　　Complications are frequent, for example side-effects of the drugs — rashes, gastro-intestinal upset, alopecia, bone-marrow depression producing anaemia and liability to superinfection.

7.　　Examples are biliary bypass for inoperable carcinoma of the head of the pancreas, intubation for inoperable carcinoma of the oesophagus, radiotherapy to localised bone secondaries, intramedullary nailing for pathological fractures, cordotomy for malignant pain in the lower limbs, transfusion for anaemia and palliative drug therapy.

8.　　Examples are anaplastic carcinoma of the thyroid, anaplastic carcinoma of the bronchus, carcinoma of the pancreas, many sarcomas.

9.　　Basal cell carcinoma of the skin, localised Hodgkin's disease, seminoma of the testis, differentiated carcinoma of the thyroid.

10.　　It was originally thought that this tumour was only 'semi-malignant' — it is rare for carcinoid tumour of the appendix to metastasise, and only 50 per cent of ileal tumours are associated with metastases.

11.　　The common example is BCG vaccination to boost the patient's immune response.

12.　　Examples of the numerous agents are nitrogen mustard, chlorambucil, 6-mercaptopurine, 5-fluorouracil, cyclophosphamide, methotrexate, vincristine, thiotepa, actinomysin D.

13.　　The breast.

14.　　The finger.

15.　　Retroperitoneal.

16.　　Examples are neuroblastoma, retinoblastoma, osteosarcoma, Wilms' tumour.

17.　　The parotid gland.

18.　　The rectus sheath.

19.　　The carotid body.

20.　　Carcinoma of skin *in situ*.

1. *Which of the following may predispose to the development of malignancy*:

(a) Exposure to 2-amino-1-naphthol
(b) Immunosuppression with azathioprine
(c) Exposure to silicone
(d) Long-standing steroid therapy
(e) Smegma

2. *The following malignancies have a better than 50 per cent five-year survival with treatment*:

(a) Papillary carcinoma of thyroid
(b) Adenocarcinoma of pancreas
(c) Seminoma of testis
(d) Hodgkin's disease
(e) Basal cell carcinoma

3. *Bone metastases are uncommon in carcinoma of the*:

(a) Prostate
(b) Lung
(c) Rectum
(d) Stomach
(e) Skin

4. *Radiotherapy is often the best primary treatment of*:

(a) Osteosarcoma
(b) Stage III carcinoma of the breast
(c) Hodgkin's disease
(d) Carcinoma of the penis
(e) Carcinoma of the colon

5. *Chemotherapy has an important role in the treatment of*:

(a) Carcinoma of the bladder

(b) Wilms' tumour
(c) Carcinoma of the cervix
(d) Seminoma
(e) Malignant effusions

Target scores U.G. 15, P.G. 20

1. (a) T Bladder tumours from aniline-dye industry
   (b) T There is an increased incidence of malignant disease
   (c) F Unlike silica
   (d) F There is no evidence of carcinogenesis
   (e) T It is thought that smegma in the uncircumcised may be a factor in carcinoma of the cervix and of the penis

2. (a) T
   (b) F
   (c) T
   (d) T
   (e) T

3. (a) F
   (b) F
   (c) T
   (d) T
   (e) T

4. (a) T
   (b) T
   (c) T After staging laparotomy
   (d) T
   (e) F

5. (a) F Although bladder instillation (for example with Epodyl) does have a small place
   (b) T Substances like actinomycin D have increased survival
   (c) F ⎫
   (d) F ⎭ Chemotherapy has little place in these conditions
   (e) T Local or systemic chemotherapy is of value in malignant pleural effusions or ascites due to carcinoma

1.   Name three serious complications of chest injury.   (2)

2.   Name three common sites of blood spread in carcinoma of the
bronchus.   (2)

3.   What is the indication for radiotherapy in bronchial carcinoma?   (2)

4.   Name three contra-indications to thoracotomy in a bronchial
carcinoma.   (2)

5.   What are the clinical features of a flail chest?   (2)

6.   What is the treatment of a flail chest?   (2)

7.   What is the mechanism of a tension pneumothorax and its
management?   (2)

8.   What are the physical signs of a coarctation of the aorta?   (2)

9.   What is the commonest cause of death in untreated aortic
coarctation?   (2)

10.   Name two benign tumours of the lung.   (2)

11.   Which is the commonest lung tumour of females?   (2)

12.   Name two hormones (or substances with hormone-like activity) that may
be secreted by lung tumours.   (3)

13.   What is a Pancoast tumour?   (3)

14.   Name two causes of bronchiectasis.   (3)

15.   Name three causes of a lung abscess.   (3)

16.   Name two complications of an empyema.   (3)

17.   What is Fallot's tetralogy?   (3)

18.   What is the percentage of five-year survivals of operable lung cancers?   (3)

19.   What is the remaining place of surgery in pulmonary tuberculosis?   (3)

20.   What is Tietze's disease?   (3)

Target Scores U.G. 21, P.G. 30, max. 49

1.   Serious complications include tension pneumothorax, flail chest, haemo-thorax, pericardial tamponade, ruptured aorta, injury to abdominal viscera.
2.   Brain, adrenals, liver and bones.

3.   In inoperable cases where there are distressing symptoms such as haemo-ptysis, pain from bone secondaries, superior vena cava obstruction, severe cough and dyspnoea from early bronchial obstruction.
4.   Scalene lymph node involvement, malignant pleural effusion, recurrent laryngeal nerve palsy, phrenic nerve paralysis, distant metastases, superior vena cava obstruction, involvement of the main pulmonary artery, very poor lung function and general condition.
5.   Dyspnoea with paradoxical movement of the chest-wall segment.
6.   First-aid procedure is to apply a pad and firm bandage. Most cases require endotracheal intubation and positive-pressure ventilation. Fixation of segment.
7.   The pleural tear has a valvular action allowing air to escape into the pleural cavity on inspiration but not to escape on expiration. Emergency treatment is to insert a wide-bore needle; definitive management requires insertion of an intercostal drain with underwater seal.
8.   Hypertension in a young adult, reduced or absent femoral pulses, large intercostal collaterals (either palpable or apparent on chest X-ray from rib erosion).
9.   Cerebral vascular accidents.

10.   Rare, but include adenomas, hamartomas, carcinoid tumour, lipomas, haemangioma.
11.   Carcinoma, which has now overtaken bronchial adenomas.
12.   Serotonin, ACTH, ADH, insulin, etc.

13.   A tumour of the lung apex which invades the brachial plexus producing severe pain.
14.   Bronchiectasis can follow any cause of bronchial obstruction associated with infection, for example pertussis, tuberculosis, foreign body, bronchial tumour.
15.   Causes include lung carcinoma, inhalation, pneumonitis or foreign body, infected cyst, infected pulmonary infarct, secondary to pneumonia or bronchiec-tasis.
16.   Bronchopleural fistula, discharge through the chest wall, septicaemia or cerebral abscess.
17.   Pulmonary stenosis, septal defect, over-riding aorta and right ventricular hypertrophy.
18.   20—30 per cent.
19.   Chronic secondary infection in a tuberculous cavity, persistent tuberculous focus in spite of adequate antituberculous treatment, tuberculous bronchiectasis.
20.   Painful non-suppurative inflammation of the costal cartilages of unknown cause, produces swelling and tenderness particularly in 1st—3rd costal cartilages.

1.   *The following features may occur in a patient with tension pneumothorax:*

(a)   Surgical emphysema
(b)   Deviation of mediastinum to the opposite side
(c)   Pulsus paradoxicus
(d)   Cyanosis

(e)   Dull percussion over pneumothorax

2.   *Which of the following procedures may be priority in a patient admitted with a flail chest:*

(a)   Immediate wiring of flail segment
(b)   Intercostal drainage of haemopneumothorax

(c)   Intubation of trachea and ventilation with respirator
(d)   Thoracotomy to exclude lung trauma
(e)   Bronchography

3.   *In carcinoma of the bronchus, which of the following statements are true:*

(a)   Adenocarcinoma is commonest
(b)   Every patient should be offered a thoracotomy
(c)   Radiotherapy should be reserved for distressing symptoms in inoperable cases
(d)   More than half are incurable at presentation
(e)   The overall prognosis is 40 per cent survival for five years

4.   *In pulmonary embolism, which of the following statements are true:*

(a)   Most patients complain of calf pain before embolus dislodged
(b)   Urgent pulmonary angiography should be routine

(c)   Venography is useful to assess chance of further major embolism
(d)   The diagnosis should be suspected if a patient develops haemoptysis after surgery
(e)   Lung scanning is the most useful investigation to establish the diagnosis

5.   *Which of the following defects should usually have surgical correction:*

(a)   Patent ductus arteriosus
(b)   Aortic incompetence
(c)   Constrictive pericarditis
(d)   Aortic coarctation
(e)   Fallot's tetralogy

Target scores U.G. 14, P.G. 20

1. (a)   T   When a rib is fractured, air may be forced into the tissue
   (b)   T   This is evidence of tension in a pneumothorax
   (c)   F
   (d)   T   Cyanosis commonly develops in a patient with a tension pneumo-
                         thorax
   (e)   F

2. (a)   F   There is no urgency for operative fixation
   (b)   T   This is an early priority if a significant volume of air and blood is
                         present
   (c)   T   Ventilation is standard procedure for severe chest injuries
   (d)   F
   (e)   F

3. (a)   F   Squamous cell carcinoma (50—60 per cent)
   (b)   F   Most patients are inoperable at diagnosis

   (c)   T   There is no benefit in giving radiotherapy to asymptomatic cases
   (d)   T   See (b)
   (e)   F   Even if tumour is resected, only 25 per cent survive five years

4. (a)   F   Many pulmonary emboli come from a silent DVT
   (b)   F   Routine pulmonary angiography is unrealistic unless embolectomy or
                         local streptokinase are considered
   (c)   T   Bilateral leg venograms should be routine after pulmonary embolism

   (d)   T   Haemoptysis after surgery is usually due to embolism
   (e)   T   Lung scans are useful to confirm the diagnosis

5. (a)   T
   (b)   F   Surgery is rarely indicated
   (c)   T
   (d)   T
   (e)   T

1. Name two causes of jaundice in neonates. (1)

2. What is the sex incidence of hypertrophic pyloric stenosis? (1)

3. What condition produces meconium ileus? (1)

4. What is the commonest congenital heart defect? (1)

5. How do you confirm the diagnosis of Hirschsprung's disease? (1)

6. What is the underlying cause of volvulus neonatorum? (2)

7. What is the commonest type of oesophageal atresia? (2)

8. What is the commonest site for a bowel atresia? (2)

9. Name two congenital anomalies of the intestine. (2)

10. What is an omphalocoele? (2)

11. What condition is detected by Ortolani's test? (2)

12. What is the commonest intestinal parasite of children in temperate zones? (2)

13. What is the presentation of eventration of the diaphragm? (2)

14. Name two malignant tumours of children. (2)

15. What percentage of biliary atresias are surgically correctable? (3)

16. Name an operation for Hirschsprung's disease. (3)

17. What is the commonest reticulosis in children? (3)

18. What are the features of the Pierre—Robin syndrome? (3)

19. Name a malignant tumour of children known to undergo spontaneous remission rarely. (3)

20. What is the prune belly syndrome? (3)

Target scores U.G. 18, P.G. 28, max. 41

1.   'Physiological' jaundice, Rhesus incompatibility, infection, hepatitis, biliary atresia.

2.   Boys four times as common as girls.

3.   Fibrocystic disease of the pancreas (mucoviscidosis).

4.   Atrial septal defect.

5.   Muscle biopsy of the rectum to show absence of ganglia.

6.   Malrotation of the gut producing a very high caecum and a narrow small-bowel mesentery.

7.   85 per cent have a blind upper pouch and a fistula between the lower oesophagus and the trachea.

8.   The duodenum.

9.   Atresia, stenosis, Meckel's diverticulum, malrotation, duplication, Hirschsprung's disease, anorectal agenesis.

10.   Defect of the peri-umbilical abdominal wall, in which the caelomic cavity is covered by peritoneum and amnium only.

11.   Congenital hip dislocation.

12.   Threadworms.

13.   Respiratory difficulty and chest infection.

14.   Neuroblastoma, nephroblastoma, retinoblastoma, osteogenic sarcoma, medulloblastoma, Ewing's sarcoma.

15.   Five per cent.

16.   Examples are Duhamel abdominoperineal pull-through, Swenson abdominoperineal pull-through, and Soave endorectal pull-through.

17.   Lymphosarcoma.

18.   Micrognathia and glossoptosis, often associated with a cleft palate.

19.   Neuroblastoma is the most frequently recorded.

20.   Congenital absence of abdominal wall muscles.

1. *A typical case of hypertrophic pyloric stenosis will:*

(a) Be a boy
(b) Have vomiting from birth
(c) Have anorexia
(d) Have a palpable mass after feeds
(e) Be satisfactorily treated with atropine methylnitrate

2. *The following congenital conditions usually require operative correction:*

(a) Congenital dislocation of hips

(b) Capillary haemangiomata
(c) Fibrocystic disease of the pancreas

(d) Congenital inguinal hernia
(e) Umbilical hernia

3. *Oesophageal atresia:*

(a) Often presents with cyanosis and regurgitation
(b) Usually responds to gentle dilatation
(c) Usually has an associated tracheal fistula
(d) Is managed with cervical oesophagostomy
(e) May be associated with anorectal agenesis

4. *Bleeding from the anus in a child may be due to:*

(a) Fissure
(b) Haemorrhoids
(c) Juvenile polyp
(d) Meckel's diverticulum
(e) Anorectal agenesis

5. *In congenital dislocation of the hip:*

(a) There may be a family history
(b) Coxa valga is common
(c) Trendelenburg's test is positive at birth

(d) Operative reduction is usual
(e) Diagnosis after two is rarely compatible with satisfactory treatment

Target scores U.G. 12, P.G. 17

1. (a) T   80 per cent are male
   (b) F   Symptoms usually do not commence for 3—4 weeks
   (c) F   The baby is hungry
   (d) T   Most cases have a palpable pylorus
   (e) F   Most cases require a Rammstedt operation

2. (a) F   CDH should normally be diagnosed early and respond to conservative
            measures
   (b) F   'Strawberry naevi' usually resolve spontaneously
   (c) F   Surgery has no place except for intestinal complications of muco-
            viscidosis
   (d) T   This rarely resolves spontaneously
   (e) F   Many cases close without surgery

3. (a) T   Due to regurgitation of saliva and feeds
   (b) F   Stenosis is rare
   (c) T   Most cases have an associated fistula
   (d) F   Primary anastomosis is the treatment of choice
   (e) T   There is a higher incidence of other anomalies

4. (a) T   This is a fairly common cause
   (b) F   Haemorrhoids are very rare in children
   (c) T   The commonest large-bowel polyp in children
   (d) T   Ectopic epithelium may ulcerate and bleed
   (e) F   Bleeding is not the presentation of this group of conditions

5. (a) T   Family history is common
   (b) T   Coxa valga is usual
   (c) F   This is a late sign — the buttock crease dips on standing on the
            affected leg
   (d) F   Occasionally operation is required to reduce the dislocation
   (e) T   Most cases are left with a limp and a tendency to osteo-arthritis later
            in life

1.   What is a Thiersch graft? (1)

2.   What is a Wolfe graft? (1)

3.   What is a pedicle graft? (1)

4.   What are two common causes of failure of skin grafts? (1)

5.   What sort of patients are most liable to keloid formation? (1)

6.   Name three malignant tumours of skin. (2)

7.   What is a rhinoplasty? (2)

8.   What is commonly used for augmentation mammoplasty? (2)

9.   What is the most useful test to distinguish between partial- and full-thickness burns? (2)

10.   What are two serious complications of burns? (2)

11.   What is the 'rule of nine'? (2)

12.   In estimating burn size, what percentage of surface area is represented by the patient's palm? (2)

13.   Name two measures to counteract infection in burns. (2)

14.   What is the management of a partial-thickness hand burn? (2)

15.   What would be an indication for Z-plasty? (2)

16.   What are the usual methods of treating a keloid scar? (2)

17.   What is the commonest facial fracture? (2)

18.   What is the name given to gastroduodenal stress ulceration in burns? (2)

19.   What percentage of surface area of burn indicates the need for intravenous therapy in adults? (3)

20.   Give an alternative name for rhytidectomy. (3)

Target scores U.G. 18, P.G. 28, max. 37

1.   Partial-thickness skin graft.

2.   Full-thickness skin graft.

3.   Full-thickness graft with subcutaneous tissue raised in stages as a tube pedicle for transferring skin to a distant site in the body.

4.   Haematoma and infection, inadequate immobilisation.

5.   Coloured races, children, and pregnant women.

6.   Squamous cell carcinoma (epithelioma), malignant melanoma, basal cell carcinoma (rodent ulcer).

7.   Operation to correct nasal deformity.

8.   Silastic implant.

9.   Partial-thickness burns retain pain sensation to pinprick.

10.   Hypovolaemia and septicaemia from secondary infection, deformity from scarring, pulmonary involvement, eye involvement.

11.   A formula to calculate the fluid requirements of a burns patient in which the surface area of the limbs and trunk, and head and neck, are divided into multiples of nine for easy calculation.

12.   One per cent.

13.   Exposure, topical antiseptics and antibiotics, systemic antibiotics.

14.   Closed management with hand dressed in position of function, and subsequent physiotherapy.

15.   A common indication is lengthening of a scar contracture line, or change in the direction of a scar.

16.   Steroid injection, excision and superficial irradiation to healing scar.

17.   Fractured zygomatic arch.

18.   Curling's ulcer.

19.   Approximately 15 per cent.

20.   Face lift.

1.   *A patient presents with a 50 per cent burn. Priority treatment would include:*

(a)   Excision and grafting
(b)   Covering burn with pig skin
(c)   Intravenous fluid therapy
(d)   Covering burnt area with dry dressings
(e)   Exposure of the burnt area

2.   *The following are common causes of serious infection in burnt patients:*

(a)   *Pseudomonas pyocyanea*
(b)   *Streptococci*
(c)   *Staphylococci*
(d)   *Clostridium welchi*
(e)   *Bacteroides*

3.   *Widely used prophylactic agents against infection or burns are:*

(a)   Penicillin powder
(b)   Sulphamylon
(c)   Silver nitrate
(d)   Tannin
(e)   Acetic acid

4.   *The following statements about skin grafts are true:*

(a)   The chance of 'take' is proportional to the graft thickness
(b)   Partial-thickness grafts can be stored for four weeks at 4 $^{\circ}$C
(c)   Full-thickness grafts give a better cosmetic result
(d)   Partial-thickness grafts tend to contract for 3–6 months
(e)   Hair growth and sweat gland function occur on partial-thickness grafts

5.   *The following are useful treatments for keloid scars:*

(a)   Triamcinolone injection
(b)   Ultraviolet light
(c)   Superficial irradiation
(d)   Prednisone orally
(e)   Dermabrasion

Target scores U.G. 14, P.G. 19

1. (a)   F   Debridement and grafting is a late priority in a burn of this extent
   (b)   F   Xenografts may be used later for dressing and for grafting
   (c)   T   This is an urgent priority
   (d)   F }   Most extensive burns are better exposed or dressed with antiseptic
   (e)   T }   solutions

2. (a)   T   This organism is a problem in a burns unit
   (b)   T   Often leading to graft failure
   (c)   T   Staphylococcal infections are also common
   (d)   F   This organism fortunately rarely colonises burns patients
   (e)   F   These anaerobic bowel organisms do not commonly infect burns

3. (a)   F   This commonly leads to hypersensitivity reactions or resistance
   (b)   T   This is useful as a cream
   (c)   T   This is effective against most common pathogens
   (d)   F   Toxic and no longer used
   (e)   F   Vinegar is not poured on burns!

4. (a)   F   Thinner grafts have more chance
   (b)   T   This is useful if grafts fail
   (c)   T   Hence are used on the face — but size is limited
   (d)   T   This may be a problem in certain sites
   (e)   F   The graft is more superfical than this

5. (a)   T   Steroid injections can soften keloid scars
   (b)   F   No value in keloids
   (c)   T   Superficial X-rays can be useful
   (d)   F   Steroids are not given orally for this condition
   (e)   F   Worse keloids are likely

1.	What is the commonest skin cyst?	(1)
2.	What is the commonest site for a rodent ulcer?	(1)
3.	What is the commonest site for a sebaceous cyst?	(1)
4.	What is the aetiology of pilonidal sinus?	(1)
5.	Where would you expect to find an onychogryphosis?	(1)
6.	What is the significance of senile keratosis?	(2)
7.	What is the difference between a sinus and a fistula?	(2)
8.	What is the initial treatment of malignant melanoma?	(2)
9.	What is the commonest subcutaneous tumour?	(2)
10.	What is the commonest congenital skin cyst?	(2)
11.	What are the skin manifestations of neurofibromatosis?	(2)
12.	Where would you expect to find an external angular dermoid?	(2)
13.	Name two common sites for squamous cell carcinoma of the skin.	(2)
14.	What is the commonest site for an implantation dermoid?	(2)
15.	What is the surgical treatment of hyperhidrosis?	(3)
16.	Where would you find glands of Montgomery?	(3)
17.	What is a rhinophyma?	(3)
18.	What is the commonest site for a molluscum sebaceum?	(3)
19.	What is the clinical significance of Campbell de Morgan spots?	(3)
20.	What are the clinical features of a glomus tumour?	(3)

Target scores U.G. 18, P.G. 28, max. 41

1.   Sebaceous cyst.

2.   Face, in the distribution of the second branch of the 5th cranial nerve.

3.   The scalp.

4.   Implantation of hairs, producing foreign body reaction and chronic sinuses.

5.   Hallux nail.

6.   It may undergo malignant change.

7.   A fistula is a tract connecting two epithelial surfaces, a sinus is a blind-ended tract.

8.   Wide excision and skin grafting. Block dissection of lymph nodes if involved.

9.   Lipoma.

10.   Dermoid cyst.

11.   Café-au-lait spots.

12.   At the lateral end of the eyebrow.

13.   Face, and dorsum of hand; that is, exposed areas.

14.   The finger.

15.   Local excision of the involved skin, or sympathectomy.

16.   The areola of the breast.

17.   Red bulbous nose due to hypertrophy of sebaceous tissues.

18.   Face and nose.

19.   None at all.

20.   Exquisitely tender little blue or reddish raised lesions, occurring in young adults, particularly the finger or nail-bed.

1. *A sebaceous cyst*:

(a) Is a variety of retention cyst

(b) Most commonly occurs in the axilla
(c) Has a lining of columnar epithelium
(d) Is not attached to skin
(e) Occasionally occurs on the palms and soles

2. *Rodent ulcers of the face are satisfactorily treated by*:

(a) Excision with a few millimetres' clearance
(b) Local radiotherapy
(c) Excision with more than a centimetre's clearance
(d) Oral 5-fluorouracil
(e) Cryosurgery

3. *In malignant melanoma*:

(a) The lesion is always deeply pigmented
(b) Hair growth is a sign of malignant change in a mole
(c) The commonest site is the face
(d) Radiotherapy is the primary treatment
(e) Monobloc prophylactic node excision is vital

4. *The following conditions predispose to squamous cell carcinoma*:

(a) Long-standing leg ulceration
(b) Lupus vulgaris
(c) Bowen's disease
(d) Exposure to radiation
(e) Exposure to β-naphthylamine

5. *The following conditions require radical surgery or radiotherapy*:

(a) Junctional naevus
(b) Capillary haemangioma
(c) Glomus tumour
(d) Kaposi sarcoma

(e) Marjolin ulcer

Target scores U.G. 14, P.G. 19

1 (a) T   Sebaceous cysts are probably caused by blocked sebaceous gland ducts
  (b) F   Scalp
  (c) F   Squamous epithelium
  (d) F   The cysts commence in the dermis and are attached to skin
  (e) F   There are no sebaceous glands in these hairless areas

2. (a) T   This is adequate clearance for these tumours
   (b) T   Radiotherapy is satisfactory for most basal cell carcinomas
   (c) F   This clearance is far too radical
   (d) F   Oral or systemic chemotherapy has no place in management
   (e) T   Cryosurgery is effective for many rodent ulcers

3. (a) F   Amelanotic lesions do occur
   (b) F   Hair growth from a malignant mole is rare
   (c) F   The leg is commoner except for lentigo maligna
   (d) F   Primary treatment is wide excision — radiotherapy is not useful
   (e) F   There is no evidence that prophylactic node dissection is useful

4. (a) T   The so-called Marjolin's ulcer
   (b) T   These TB lesions can turn malignant
   (c) T   This is carcinoma-in-situ of skin
   (d) T   Many pioneers with X-rays developed skin cancer
   (e) F   This may produce bladder cancer but not skin cancer

5. (a) F   This is benign
   (b) F   Strawberry naevus — best left alone
   (c) F   This acutely painful lesion of blood vessels is benign
   (d) T   Multicentre malignant tumour of blood vessels and fibroblasts, commoner in Africa
   (e) T   See 4(a)

1.   What is Bell's palsy?   (1)

2.   Name three causes of epistaxis.   (1)

3,   What would be an indication for myringotomy?   (1)
4.   Name three causes of deafness.   (1)

5.   What are the symptoms of Ménière's syndrome?   (1)
6.   What is the treatment of Ménière's syndrome?   (1)
7.   What would be an indication for a Caldwell Luc operation?   (2)
8.   What is a myringoplasty?   (2)
9.   What is Rinné's test?   (2)

10.   What is otosclerosis?   (2)

11.   What is the usual treatment of otosclerosis?   (2)
12.   What would be an indication for a nasal septoplasty?   (2)
13.   What are singers' nodes?   (2)

14.   What is the treatment of carcinoma localised in the vocal cord?   (2)

15.   Name three causes of hoarseness.   (3)

16.   What is the commonest cause of tracheal stenosis?   (3)

17.   What is a cholesteatoma?   (3)

18.   What is an internal auditory meatus tumour?   (3)

19.   What is a glomus jugulare tumour?   (3)

20.   What is a torus palatinus?   (3)

Target scores U.G. 18, P.G. 27, max. 40

1.   Acute facial nerve palsy of unknown aetiology, possibly due to nerve oedema during its course in the base of the skull.

2.   Many causes include: local lesions — trauma, nasal polyps, nasal tumours, antral tumours, etc.; general causes — hypertension, bleeding diseases (for example anticoagulants), thrombocytopenic purpura, leukaemia.

3.   Severe acute otitis media with pus in the middle ear.

4.   Conductive causes such as wax in external auditory meatus, perforation of the eardrum, chronic otitis media, tympanic perforations, otosclerosis, ossicula chain disruption, middle ear adhesions. Neural causes include advancing age, trauma, viral bacterial infections, Ménière's syndrome, diabetes, vascular obstruction.

5.   Neural deafness, tinnitus and vertigo, with vomiting.

6.   Stemetil; in severe cases, destruction of the labyrinth.

7.   Purulent maxillary sinusitis, severe, acute or recurrent.

8.   Repair of a perforated eardrum.

9.   Tuning fork vibrated firstly lateral to the ear and then on the mastoid to differentiate conduction deafness from nerve deafness.

10.   Progressive conductive hearing loss dates from puberty or after without evidence of eardrum or middle-ear disease. Stapes becomes fixed.

11.   Stapedectomy and replacement with prosthesis.

12.   Deviated septum causing nasal obstruction.

13.   Tiny projections from the free edge of the cord resembling a grain of sand, usually at the juncture of the anterior and middle thirds, caused by singing or shouting.

14.   Radiotherapy. If tumour persists or recurs but is still confined laryngectomy may be indicated.

15.   Causes include acute and chronic laryngitis, singers' nodules, granulomas, polyps of the vocal cord, papilloma of the larynx, tumours of the larynx, laryngeal paralysis.

16.   Endotracheal intubation or tracheostomy with prolonged inflation of the cuff.

17.   Squamous epithelial sac that has grown inward from the skin of the ear canal or drum, tends to enlarge gradually and may erode the bone surrounding the antrum and give rise to meningitis or brain abscess.

18.   A schwannoma — a benign tumour of the sheath of the 8th nerve. Tends to erode the bone and eventually produces 7th and 8th nerve palsies.

19.   Vascular tumour arising from the jugular bulb and spreading upward into the middle ear space and posteriorly into the mastoid gland. Eventually produces paralysis of cranial nerves 9, 10, 11, and then 7, 8 and 12.

20.   Palatal exostosis — bony submucosal nodules projecting down from the middle of the hard palate.

1.   *Common causes of nasal airway obstruction are*:

(a)   Rhinophyma

(b)   Vasomotor rhinitis
(c)   Deviated septum
(d)   Juvenile angiofibroma
(e)   Nasal carcinoma

2.   *In patients with epistaxis*:

(a)   A blood dyscrasia causes the bleeding in five per cent of cases

(b)   Most cases require diathermy to the bleeding point
(c)   The bleeding point is usually near the nares
(d)   Bleeding from the posterior nose usually requires anterior and posterior
        packing
(e)   Main artery ligation can be necessary

3.   *Neural deafness may be due to*:

(a)   Diabetes
(b)   Vascular disease
(c)   Otosclerosis
(d)   Chronic otitis media
(e)   Acoustic neuroma

4.   *Acute otitis media*:

(a)   Is commonest in the second decade
(b)   Usually presents with ear discharge
(c)   Often leads to permanent deafness
(d)   May require myringotomy
(e)   Is usually precipitated by upper respiratory tract infection

5.   *Carcinoma of the larynx*:

(a)   95 per cent are squamous cell carcinomas
(b)   Presents with stridor
(c)   Early diagnosis is compatible with conservation of the voice
(d)   Primary treatment is usually radiation
(e)   Subglottic lesions usually require laryngectomy

Target scores U.G. 13, P.G. 18

1. (a) F   This is swelling of the nasal skin from connective tissue and glandular hyperplasia
   (b) T   Hay fever leads to mucosal congestion as well as excess secretions
   (c) T   Septal deviation is a common cause of blocked nose
   (d) F   This is a rare tumour in teenage boys
   (e) F   Rare

2. (a) F   Although a blood disorder may present with epistaxis, very few cases are due to this
   (b) F   Most cases stop spontaneously or with compression
   (c) T   Sometimes called Littre's area or Kiesselbach's triangle
   (d) T   After local anaesthesia and vasoconstriction has been applied
   (e) T   Rarely packing fails and ligation of anterior ethmoid, internal maxillary or external carotid is required

3. (a) T ⎫
   (b) T ⎬ Both these conditions may be present in the ageing
   (c) F ⎫
   (d) F ⎬ These would be conductive causes
   (e) T   Most patients with an acoustic neuroma have unilateral hearing loss

4. (a) F   Children are commonly affected
   (b) F   Only if drum has ruptured. Pain and acute deafness are commoner
   (c) F   This is fortunately rare
   (d) T   If severely painful bulging tympanic membrane is apparent
   (e) T   Causing blockage of the eustachian tube

5. (a) T
   (b) F   Hoarseness and pain. Airway obstruction is late
   (c) T   With radiotherapy and/or partial laryngectomy
   (d) T   If confined to true vocal cord often 6000 rads are given
   (e) T   If the lesion extends more than 1 cm below the free edge of the cord

1. What is the commonest carcinoma of the female reproductive tract? (1)
2. What is the pathological name for 'fibroids'? (1)
3. What is the commonest treatment for carcinoma of the cervix? (1)
4. What is the commonest pathological type of carcinoma of the cervix? (1)
5. Name three congenital anomalies of the uterus and vagina. (2)

6. What two organisms commonly cause vaginitis? (2)
7. What are the common extra-uterine sites for endometriosis? (2)
8. What are the typical clinical features of an ectopic pregnancy? (2)

9. Name two causes of a vesicovaginal fistula. (2)

10. What is the commonest cause of infertility in the female? (2)
11. Where does a Bartholin's abscess present? (2)
12. Name two symptoms of fibroids. (2)

13. Name two complications of ovarian cysts. (2)
14. Name three types of ovarian cysts. (3)

15. How do the presenting features differ in carcinoma of the body of the uterus and carcinoma of the cervix? (3)

16. Name two complications of carcinoma of the cervix. (3)

17. How is carcinoma of the cervix staged? (3)

18. Name three clinical features of endometriosis. (3)

19. How does a hydatidiform mole usually present? (3)
20. What is the mainstay of treatment of choriocarcinoma (3)

Target scores U.G. 17, P.G. 26, max. 43

1.   Carcinoma of the cervix.
2.   Leiomyomas.
3.   Radiotherapy.
4.   Squamous cell carcinoma.
5.   Imperforate hymen, duplication of the vagina, transverse vaginal septum, absent vagina, bicornuate uterus, are examples. Many cases of imperfect development are associated with intersex states.
6.   *Trichomonas* and monilial infections.
7.   Ovaries, pouch of Douglas, uterosacral ligaments and rectovaginal septum.
8.   Missed period with possible symptoms of pregnancy, vaginal bleeding, lower abdominal colic which may become generalised with shock and referred pain to the shoulder. Widespread abdominal tenderness, slightly enlarged uterus, tender forniceal mass.
9.   Causes include impaction of the foetal head, radiotherapy or damage to the urinary tract during pelvic surgery.
10.   Chronic salpingitis.
11.   Posterior labia majora.
12.   Abnormal uterine bleeding, vague pelvic discomfort or pressure on neighbouring organs, for example frequency, constipation. Sudden pain from degeneration or torsion. Infertility and obstructed labour.
13.   Haemorrhage into cyst, torsion, malignant change, rupture, infection.
14.   Follicular cyst, corpus luteum cyst, dermoid cyst, cystic tumours (for example cystadenoma, cystadenocarcinomas), endometrial (chocolate) cysts.
15.   Carcinoma of the uterus occurs in the older age group and usually presents with post-menopausal bleeding. Carcinoma of the cervix occurs between the ages of 40 and 50 and presents with vaginal discharge and intermenstrual bleeding.
16.   Complications include obstruction to the ureter producing hydronephrosis and uraemia if bilateral, lymphoedema, invasion of lumbosacral plexus, vesicovaginal fistula, rectovaginal fistula; blood loss may lead to anaemia.
17.   Stage 0: carcinoma *in situ*; stage 1: confined to the cervix; stage 2: extended beyond the cervix but not to the pelvic wall or lower third of the vagina; stage 3: extending to the lower third of the vagina or pelvic wall; stage 4: extending beyond the true pelvis or involving the mucosa of bladder or rectum.
18.   Features include pain before and during menstruation, may be accompanied by dyspareunia and rectal tenesmus, continuous vague lower abdominal and pelvic discomfort exaggerated during menstruation, low back pain, painful defaecation associated with menstrual period, irregular periods, dysuria, large-bowel colic. Examination showing tender pelvic nodules of endometriosis; bilateral tender fixed ovarian cystic masses may be felt.
19.   Like a threatened abortion.
20.   Chemotherapy, for example methotrexate.

1. *Relatively common malignant ovarian tumours are:*

(a) Dysgerminoma
(b) Arrhenoblastoma
(c) Cystadenocarcinoma
(d) Undifferentiated adenocarcinoma
(e) Krukenberg tumour

2. *Cancer of the cervix:*

(a) Is more common than carcinoma of breast in the UK
(b) The incidence is related to sexual activity

(c) Is commonest between the ages of 40 and 50
(d) Lymph node metastasis is not related to extent of local spread
(e) Often presents with intermenstrual or post-coital bleeding

3. *Endometriosis:*

(a) Is commonest in the elderly
(b) Is more common in the infertile
(c) Often presents with dysmenorrhoea
(d) Most cases have irregular periods
(e) Most cases require surgical excision

4. *The clinical features of a patient with a ruptured ectopic pregnancy may include:*

(a) No history of menstrual disturbance
(b) Bluish discoloration around the umbilicus
(c) Shoulder pain
(d) Vaginal bleeding
(e) A past history of infertility or salpingitis

5. *Leiomyomas of the uterus:*

(a) Are rarely asymptomatic
(b) Occur in 20 per cent of Western women
(c) Turn malignant in five per cent of cases
(d) Are the commonest indication for hysterectomy
(e) Do not give rise to pain

Target scores U.G. 10, P.G. 15

1. (a) F   This is a rare tumour of germ cell origin
   (b) F   A rare tumour producing masculinisation
   (c) T   Serous and mucous types are common
   (d) T
   (e) F   This is transcoelomic spread from gastro-intestinal cancer

2. (a) F   Carcinoma of the breast is more common
   (b) T   The condition is more common among the sexually active and
            promiscuous
   (c) T   Compare carcinoma *in situ* which is a decade earlier
   (d) F   Lymphatic spread corresponds fairly well to degree of local invasion
   (e) T   Often these are the first symptoms

3. (a) F   It is confined to reproductive period
   (b) T   Many patients are nulliparous or infertile
   (c) T   This is often the first symptom
   (d) F   Menstrual aberrations only occur in 50 per cent of cases
   (e) F   Hormonal treatment controls most cases

4. (a) T   A missed period is not vital to diagnosis
   (b) T   Though a rare sign — Cullen's sign
   (c) T   Due to diaphragmatic irritation by free blood
   (d) T   Vaginal bleeding may precede rupture
   (e) T   Ectopic pregnancy is more common in chronic pelvic disease

5. (a) F   They are commonly symptomless
   (b) T   And are more common in coloured races
   (c) F   Sarcomatous change is very rare
   (d) T
   (e) F   Although uncommon pain can occur, for example from degeneration
            and torsion

1.   What is the common presentation of *Schistosoma haematobium*
infection?   (1)

2.   What are the two types of leprosy?   (1)

3.   What is the common clinical effect of filariasis?   (1)

4.   What is the commonest cause of anaemia in the tropics?   (1)

5.   What is the surgical relevance of sickle-cell disease?   (2)

6.   What is the medical treatment of amoebiasis?   (2)

7.   Name two complications of ascariasis.   (2)

8.   Name a surgical complication of typhoid fever.   (2)

9.   What is the treatment of a keloid scar?   (2)

10.   What is the clinical interest of Burkitt's lymphoma?   (2)

11.   What is the commonest site for a Burkitt's lymphoma?   (2)

12.   What is the commonest cause of splenomegaly in the tropics? (2)

13.   What is the commonest cause of intestinal obstruction in the tropics? (2)

14.   What is the commonest cause of paraplegia in the tropics?   (3)

15.   What is the commonest site for a mycetoma?   (3)

16.   What is the bacteriology of a tropical ulcer?   (3)

17.   What is the most serious effect of onchocerciasis?   (3)

18.   Name two features to distinguish ileocaecal tuberculosis from
Crohn's disease.   (3)

19.   What is the common site for a Kaposi sarcoma?   (3)

20.   What are the clinical features of ainhum?   (3)

Target scores U.G. 17, P.G. 28, max. 43

1.   Haematuria.

2.   Lepromatous and tuberculoid.

3.   Lymphoedema.

4.   Hookworm infestation of the intestine.

5.   Danger of sickle-cell crisis if fall in oxygen tension during anaesthesia. May also produce micro-infarctions in the mesenteric circulation presenting as an acute abdomen. Bone infarction may predispose to osteomyelitis (frequently due to *Salmonella*), fractures and deformity (of the femoral head, for example).

6.   Metronidazole (Flagyl).

7.   Intestinal obstruction, perforation or volvulus; obstructive jaundice, rarely appendicitis, cholecystitis.

8.   Small-bowel perforation. Intestinal haemorrhage, urinary retention, cholecystitis.

9.   Triamcinolone injection or ointment, excision and injection of steroids into wound edges, or superficial X-rays.

10.   There is good evidence that this malignant tumour is due to a virus transmitted by an insect.

11.   The face.

12.   Malaria. Second most common is schistosomiasis.

13.   Strangulated hernia.

14.   Tuberculosis.

15.   Foot.

16.   Common organisms are *Fusiformis fusiformis* and *Borrelia vincenti*.

17.   Blindness.

18.   Tuberculosis affects the caecum and ascending colon, Crohn's disease usually does not. Demonstration of acid-fast bacilli, Mantoux reaction positive in tuberculosis, it may be negative in Crohn's disease. Skip lesions may be present in Crohn's disease.

19.   The limbs.

20.   Constricting ringlike lesions involving the toes and commonly leading to auto-amputation.

1. *Sickle-cell disease*:

(a) Is confined to negroes
(b) Is due to the presence of haemoglobin-T
(c) A patient with sickle-cell trait has a relative resistance to falciparum malaria in childhood
(d) Is characterised by anaemia and episodes of severe pain

(e) Is treated by ammonium chloride

2. *The following parasites can infest the human intestine*:

(a) *Entamoeba histolytica*
(b) *Taenia echinococcus*
(c) *Taenia solium*
(d) *Taenia espirantinum*
(e) *Plasmodium falciparum*

3. *Complications of malaria include*:

(a) Passage of dark-red or black urine
(b) Splenomegaly
(c) Coma
(d) Nephrotic syndrome
(e) Blindness

4. *In a patient with lepromatous leprosy*:

(a) Organisms are rarely demonstrable
(b) No cell-mediated immunity is found
(c) Skin lesions are less distinct than in the tuberculoid form
(d) Testicular atrophy may occur
(e) Nerve damage is early

5. *Burkitt's lymphoma*:

(a) Is commonest in the third and fourth decades

(b) Most frequently presents with a tumour of the mandible or maxilla
(c) Is primarily a disease of lymph nodes
(d) May present with acute paraplegia
(e) Responds poorly to chemotherapy

Target scores U.G. 19, P.G. 14

1. (a) F   Other races can be affected to a lesser extent
   (b) F   The abnormal haemoglobin is known as haemoglobin S

   (c) T   Hence the selective continuance of the inherited disease
   (d) T   Infarction crises are common, particularly affecting the spleen and
            bones
   (e) F   There is no satisfactory long-term treatment, although sodium
            bicarbonate can help alter blood pH for short periods.

2. (a) T   Amoebiasis
   (b) F   Hydatid is not primarily an intestinal infestation in man
   (c) T   Pork tape-worm
   (d) F   There is no such parasite!
   (e) F   This is a malarial parasite

3. (a) T   Due to severe intravascular haemolysis ('blackwater fever')
   (b) T   This is almost universal in endemic areas
   (c) T   Often due to cerebral falciparum malaria
   (d) T   *Plasmodium malariae* can produce immune complex nephritis
   (e) F   This is not a complication of malaria

4. (a) F   This is the infective form of the disease
   (b) T   Unlike the tuberculoid form
   (c) T   Hence the most infective form of the disease presents later
   (d) T   Often with the development of gynaecomastia
   (e) F   Nerve damage is late in this form of the disease

5. (a) F   The peak incidence is between four and eight years' old and is rare after
            puberty
   (b) T   The first clinical sign is loosening of the back teeth
   (c) F   Lymph nodes are rarely involved
   (d) T   This occurs without evidence of radiological collapse
   (e) F   Response to chemotherapy is often dramatic

1. Name a drug combination commonly used for premedication. (1)

2. What diet is useful for patients with diverticular disease? (1)

3. Name a useful post-operative anti-emetic. (1)

4. What is Vivonex an example of? (1)

5. What is the usual drug of choice for penicillin-resistant *Staphylococci*? (1)

6. Why is morphine contra-indicated in severe biliary and pancreatic pain? (1)

7. Name a drug shown to heal gastric ulcers. (2)

8. What is the commonest treatment for malaria? (2)

9. Name a drug useful for the rapid control of a thyrotoxic crisis. (2)

10. Name a drug useful in the treatment of monilial infections. (2)

11. Name a drug useful in treating gout. (2)

12. Name an antibiotic commonly implicated in the condition of pseudo-membranous colitis. (2)

13. Name an antibacterial for treatment of infection of the urinary tract but ineffective for treatment elsewhere. (2)

14. Name an antithyroid drug. (2)

15. Name a substance useful for the injection of haemorrhoids. (2)

16. Name a drug useful in the treatment of trigeminal neuralgia. (3)

17. What would be an indication for giving a patient streptokinase? (3)

18. Name a drug that is useful in prophylaxis against further attacks of ulcerative colitis. (3)

19. What is the most valuable drug for the treatment of *Bacteroides*? (3)

20. Name a use for cholestyramine. (3)

Target scores U.G. 18, P.G. 18, max. 39

1.   Pethidine and atropine, or omnopon and scopolamine.

2.   High-residue diet.

3.   Examples are prochlorperazine (Stemetil), cyclizine, metoclopramide (Maxolon), perphenazine (Fentazin).

4.   A synthetic diet producing minimal residue.

5.   Cloxacillin or flucloxacillin.

6.   Morphine produces contracture of the sphincter of Oddi.

7.   Carbenoxolone, cimetidine.

8.   Chloroquine.

9.   A beta-blocker such as propanolol.

10.   Nystatin, gentian violet.

11.   Allopurinol, phenylbutazone, probenecid, sulphinpyrazone, colchicine and aspirin.

12.   Lincomycin and clindamycin.

13.   Examples are nitrofurantoin (Furadantin) and carfecillin (Uticillin). Acidification with acid salts or mandelic acid can have antibacterial activity.

14.   Carbimazol, potassium perchlorate, thiouracil.

15.   An oily solution such as phenol in almond oil.

16.   Carbamazepine (Tegretol), clonazepan.

17.   Deep vein thrombosis and pulmonary embolism.

18.   Salazopyrin.

19.   Metronidazole (Flagyl).

20.   Cholestyramine binds bile salts and may help itching in malignant obstructive jaundice or in cases of diarrhoea when bile salts are implicated. The drug may be of value in hyperlipidaemia and hyperoxaluria.

1.   *The following drugs may be useful for preparation of the bowel for colonic surgery*:

(a)   Metronidazole
(b)   Nitrofurantoin
(c)   Magnesium sulphate
(d)   Salazopyrin
(e)   Kaolin and morphine

2.   *The following drugs are likely to be effective in Gram-negative septicaemia*:

(a)   Cloxacillin
(b)   Penicillin
(c)   Gentamycin
(d)   Erythromycin
(e)   Cephaloridine

3.   *The following drugs may be beneficial in acute pancreatitis*:

(a)   Glucagon

(b)   Calcium gluconate
(c)   Aprotinin
(d)   Calciferol
(e)   Pancreozymin

4.   *Which of these drugs may be useful in a thyrotoxic patient*:

(a)   Potassium iodide
(b)   Thyroxine
(c)   Propanolol
(d)   Potassium tetrachlorate
(e)   Carbimazole

5.   *Which of the following are useful drugs in gastro-intestinal disorders*:

(a)   Metoclopramide
(b)   Mebeverine
(c)   Cimetidine
(d)   Pancreofusan
(e)   Salazopyrin

Target scores U.G. 16, P.G. 21

1. (a)   T   Flagyl is effective against *Bacteroides* in the gut
   (b)   F   No value in bowel preparation — useful against urinary pathogens
   (c)   T   Standard oral preparation to produce diarrhoea
   (d)   F   This has anti-inflammatory action in ulcerative colitis
   (e)   F   This antidiarrhoea preparation would be undesirable in bowel preparation

2. (a)   F ⎫
   (b)   F ⎬ These drugs are ineffective against most Gram-negative infections
   (c)   T
   (d)   F   Similar spectrum to (a) and (b)
   (e)   T

3. (a)   T   Glucagon reduces pancreatic exocrine secretion and may drastically reduce pain
   (b)   T   This is for correction of hypocalcaemia in severe cases
   (c)   T   Trasylol may be effective in reducing mortality in the older patient
   (d)   F ⎫ No value in pancreatitis
   (e)   F ⎭

4. (a)   T   Particularly in preparation for surgery — but short-acting
   (b)   F
   (c)   T   Beta-blockers rapidly control symptoms and cardiovascular complication
   (d)   F   No such drug — potassium perchlorate is sometimes used
   (e)   T   Standard antithyroid drug (Neomercazole)

5. (a)   T   Promotes gastric emptying and is an anti-emetic
   (b)   T   Useful antispasmodic
   (c)   T   Tagamet — an H_2 receptor antagonist
   (d)   F   No such drug exists
   (e)   T   Useful in ulcerative colitis

1. Give three causes of uraemia. (1)

2. Name two causes of a low protein-bound iodine or serum thyroxine. (1)
3. Name two causes of marked proteinuria. (1)

4. Name two causes of hyperamylasaemia. (2)

5. Give two causes of hyponatraemia. (2)

6. Name two causes of high haemoglobin. (2)

7. Give two causes of hypo-albuminaemia. (2)

8. Give two causes of hypercapnia. (2)

9. Name two causes of a raised CSF protein. (2)
10. Give two causes of increased faecal fats. (2)

11. Give two causes of hyperkalaemia. (2)
12. Name two causes of a very high ESR. (2)
13. Give two causes of a raised SGOT. (2)

14. Give two causes of a prolonged prothrombin time. (2)
15. Name three causes of hypercalciuria. (3)

16. Give two causes of hypocalcaemia. (3)
17. Name two causes of a high blood cholesterol. (3)

18. Give two causes of a raised serum urate. (3)
19. Give two causes of hypoglycaemia. (3)
20. Give two causes of a raised serum acid phosphatase. (3)

Target scores U.G. 21, P.G. 28, max. 43

1.   Pre-renal causes such as dehydration. Renal causes such as glomerulone-phritis, chronic pyelonephritis. Post-renal causes such as prostatic hyperplasia, or any obstructive uropathy.

2.   Hypothyroidism, as in cretinism, myxoedema, Hashimoto's thyroiditis.

3.   Causes include nephrotic syndrome (massive proteinuria), glomerulone-phritis, pyelonephritis, Fanconi syndrome, analgesic nephropathy, diabetic nephropathy.

4.   Acute pancreatitis, pancreatic trauma, acute parotitis, intestinal obstruction, perforated peptic ulcer, ruptured aneurysm, ruptured ectopic pregnancy.

5.   Gastro-intestinal losses, such as chronic vomiting, diarrhoea, or intestinal obstruction. Addison's disease. Prolonged sweating and long use of diuretics or salt-free diet (assuming normal fluid intake); inappropriate ADH secretion.

6.   Polycythaemia rubra vera, chronic bronchitis and emphysema, dehydration, hypernephroma may stimulate erythropoiesis, Cushing's disease.

7.   Any severe chronic illness, such as malignant disease. Any cause of excess loss of protein, such as protein-losing enteropathy, nephrotic syndrome, failure to synthesise albumin as in liver disease, etc.

8.   Hypercapnia occurs mainly in those forms of respiratory failure in which there is inadequate gas exchange at alveoli; for example, respiratory paralysis by poliomyelitis, drugs, airway obstruction as in bronchitis and asthma.

9.   Meningitis, encephalitis, brain and spinal cord tumours.

10.   Any cause of malabsorption, such as chronic pancreatitis, obstructive jaundice, coeliac disease, small-bowel resection, or Crohn's disease.

11.   Renal failure, over-infusion of potassium, severe injury or infection.

12.   Examples are any collagen disease, such as SLE, multiple myeloma.

13.   Hepatocellular damage, for example hepatitis, drugs (chlorpromazine), poisons (phosphorus); myocardial infarction; prolonged obstructive jaundice.

14.   Liver damage; obstructive jaundice; anticoagulants.

15.   Hyperparathyroidism, sarcoidosis, milk-alkali syndrome, vitamin D intoxication, bony metastases, immobilisation.

16.   Hypoparathyroidism, severe diarrhoea, chronic renal insufficiency, rickets.

17.   Familial hypercholesterolaemia, myxoedema, nephrotic syndrome, obstructive jaundice, diabetes.

18.   Gout, renal failure, leukaemia.

19.   Insulin overdose, insulinoma, reactive (e.g. after gastrectomy).

20.   Prostatic carcinoma, rectal examination, haemolysis, occasionally in acute myelocytic leukaemia.

1.   *A raised serum amylase may be found in:*

(a)   Acute appendicitis
(b)   Acute sialadenitis
(c)   Perforated peptic ulcer
(d)   Acute prostatitis
(e)   Polycystic kidneys

2.   *Hypercalcaemia may occur in:*

(a)   Bone metastases
(b)   Hypoparathyroidism
(c)   Sarcoidosis
(d)   Parathyroid tumours
(e)   Renal failure

3.   *Hyperkalaemia may be caused by:*

(a)   Conn's syndrome
(b)   Renal failure
(c)   Burns
(d)   Crush injury
(e)   Intestinal obstruction

4.   *A low serum magnesium may be due to:*

(a)   Malabsorption
(b)   Primary hyperaldosteronism
(c)   Hypoparathyroidism
(d)   Hypothyroidism
(e)   Hypersplenism

5.   *The following investigations may be abnormal in liver disease:*

(a)   Prothrombin time
(b)   Albumin
(c)   Alpha-fetoprotein
(d)   Acid phosphatase
(e)   Serum ammonia

Target scores U.G. 14, P.G. 19

1. (a)   F
   (h)   T   Any inflammatory process in salivary glands
   (c)   T   Possibly due to absorption of pancreatic amylase from the peritoneum
   (d)   F
   (e)   F

2. (a)   T
   (b)   F   Hyperparathyroidism
   (c)   T
   (d)   T   Most cases of hyperparathyroidism
   (e)   T   Secondary hyperparathyroidism can occur

3. (a)   F   Hypokalaemia is usual
   (b)   T   This is the commonest cause
   (c)   T   Due to excessive release of cellular potassium
   (d)   T   As for (c)
   (e)   F   Hypokalaemia is more likely

4. (a)   T   And any prolonged diarrhoea or starvation
   (b)   T
   (c)   T   Particularly when large doses of calcium and vitamin D are required
   (d)   F
   (e)   F

5. (a)   T
   (b)   T   Albumin levels are often low in chronic liver disease
   (c)   T   This abnormal protein may be found in hepatoma
   (d)   F   This is raised in prostatic carcinoma
   (e)   T   Serum ammonia levels may be raised in portal hypertension due to
              cirrhosis

1.   Name a branch of the common carotid artery before its division into internal and external carotid arteries.   (1)
2.   What are the contents of the carotid sheath?   (1)
3.   What muscles form the anterior abdominal wall?   (1)
4.   Name four carpal bones.   (1)

5.   From which artery does the cystic artery normally arise?   (1)
6.   On which muscle does the phrenic nerve descend to the thoracic inlet?   (2)
7.   Name four constituents of the spermatic cord.   (2)

8.   Name the arterial supply to the colon.   (2)

9.   Which muscles give rise to the conjoint tendon, and what is the nerve supply in that region?   (2)
10.   Name five muscles acting on the shoulder joint.   (2)

11.   Name three branches of the internal iliac artery.   (2)

12.   Name four structures that pierce the diaphragm.   (2)

13.   Name the arterial supply to the thyroid with the origin of the arteries.   (2)

14.   Name three branches of the external carotid artery.   (2)

15.   Name three muscles supplied by the obturator nerve.   (3)

16.   What are the relations of the femoral ring?   (3)

17.   Name three muscles attached to the clavicle.   (3)

18.   What structures lie to the front and back of the epiploic foramen of Winslow?   (3)
19.   Name five divisions of the right bronchus.   (3)

20.   What is the distribution of the ulnar nerve in the hand?   (3)

Target scores U.G. 17, P.G. 26, max. 41

1.   There are none!

2.   Internal and common carotid arteries, internal jugular vein, vagus nerve.
3.   Rectus abdominis, external and internal oblique, transversus abdominis.
4.   Proximal row — scaphoid, lunate, triquetrum, pisiform. Distal row —
trapezium, trapezoid, capitate, hamate.
5.   Right hepatic artery.
6.   Scalenus anterior.

7.   Processus vaginalis, vas deferens with nerves and vessels, testicular artery,
nerves and lymphatics, areolar tissue, pampiniform plexus, spermatic fascias, crema-
steric muscle with vessels and nerves.
8.   Ileocolic, right colic, middle colic (branches of superior mesenteric artery),
left colic and sigmoid (branches of inferior mesenteric artery).
9.   Internal oblique and transversus abdominis; L1 via ilio-inguinal and genitofemoral nerves.
10.   Supraspinatus, infraspinatus, teres major and minor, subscapularis, pectoralis major, latissimus dorsi and rhomboids, long head of triceps. Not primarily
acting on shoulder joint but on pectoral girdle are trapezius, levator scapulae,
serratus anterior and pectoralis minor.
11.   Umbilical, superior and inferior vesical, middle rectal, superior and inferior gluteal, obturator, internal pudendal, iliolumbar and lateral sacral arteries.
12.   Inferior vena cava, oesophagus, aorta, branches of phrenic nerves, vagal
trunks, thoracic duct, splanchnic nerves.
13.   Superior thyroid artery (branch of external carotid), inferior thyroid
artery (branch of thyrocervical trunk of subclavian), occasional thyroidea ima
artery (from aorta or other main arteries).
14.   Superior thyroid, ascending pharyngeal, lingual, facial, occipital, posterior
auricular, maxillary, and superficial temporal.
15.   The adductors — brevis, longus, magnus, gracilis, obturator externus and
occasionally pectineus.
16.   Lateral — femoral vein; medial — lacunar ligament; posterior — pubis with
pectineal ligament and pectineus fascia; anterior — inguinal ligament.
17.   Trapezius, deltoid, sternomastoid, pectoralis major, subclavius and sterno-
hyoid.
18.   Anteriorly — common bile duct, hepatic artery, portal vein. Posteriorly —
inferior vena cava.
19.   There are ten: upper lobe — apical, posterior, anterior; middle lobe —
lateral and medial; lower lobe — superior, anterior basal, medial basal, lateral basal,
posterior basal.
20.   Sensory — medial 1½ fingers; all short muscles of the hand except lateral
two lumbricals and thenar muscles.

1.   *The following arteries are part of the Circle of Willis*:

(a)   Posterior communicating
(b)   Anterior cerebral
(c)   Middle communicating
(d)   Posterior cerebral
(e)   Vertebral

2.   *The following would be paralysed in a complete ulnar nerve injury at the elbow*:

(a)   Pronator teres
(b)   Thenar muscles
(c)   Flexor carpi ulnaris
(d)   Adductor pollicis
(e)   Interossei

3.   *The ureter crosses the following structures*:

(a)   Genitofemoral nerve
(b)   Iliac arteries
(c)   Psoas major
(d)   Thoracic duct
(e)   Sympathetic chain

4.   *The following structures are intimately related to the first rib*:

(a)   Carotid body
(b)   Stellate ganglion
(c)   Pleura
(d)   Vertebral artery
(e)   Hypoglossal nerve

5.   *The following statements about the oesophagus are correct*:

(a)   In an adult it measures 10 cm
(b)   It is closely related to the arch of the vena azygos
(c)   It is a smooth muscle tube
(d)   The nerve supply is from T1—8 intercostal nerves
(e)   Mucous glands are absent in the oesophagus

Target scores U.G. 10, P.G. 15

1. (a)   T
   (b)   T
   (c)   F   There is no such artery
   (d)   T
   (e)   F   The vertebrals join to form the basilar artery which divides into the posterior cerebral arteries

2. (a)   F ⎫
   (b)   F ⎬ These are supplied by the median nerve
   (c)   T
   (d)   T
   (e)   T

3. (a)   T
   (b)   T   Either the common or beginning external iliacs
   (c)   T   The ureter runs down and crosses the muscle
   (d)   F
   (e)   F

4. (a)   F
   (b)   T   Near neck of first rib
   (c)   T   The lung apex emerges from the thoracic inlet
   (d)   T   First branch of the subclavian artery
   (e)   F

5. (a)   F   10" (25 cm)
   (b)   T
   (c)   F   The upper two-thirds contain striated muscle
   (d)   F   Vagus and sympathetic nerves
   (e)   F   Racemose mucous glands are found

1.   Name two operations for ulcerative colitis.   (1)

2.   What is the commonest shunt performed for portal hypertension?   (1)
3.   Name three approaches for prostatectomy.   (1)
4.   Which abdominal branches of the vagus nerve are preserved in a
highly selective vagotomy?   (1)
5.   Name three operations in the primary treatment of early breast   (1)
cancer.
6.   Whose name is attached to the commonest operation for hallux   (1)
valgus?
7.   What is the commonest method of arterial embolectomy?   (1)
8.   Give an alternative name for a Rammstedt operation.   (1)
9.   Name three approaches to a femoral hernia repair.   (2)

10.   What structures are removed in a Whipple's operation?   (2)

11.   Describe two methods of removing a common duct stone.   (2)

12.   What is the best approach for draining a subphrenic abscess?   (2)
13.   What is the first structure to be divided when doing an emergency
splenectomy?   (2)
14.   What is the commonest operation for idiopathic hydronephrosis?   (2)
15.   Give three indications for adrenalectomy.   (3)

16.   Give four sites or types of lower-limb amputation.   (3)

17.   Name two indications for pulmonary lobectomy.   (3)

18.   Name three approaches to a cervical sympathectomy.   (3)

19.   Which ganglia should be removed in a lumbar sympathectomy?   (3)
20.   Name two operations for complete rectal prolapse.   (3)

Target scores U.G. 16, P.G. 26, max. 38

1.   Panproctocolectomy and ileostomy; total colectomy and ileorectal anastomosis.

2.   Portocaval.

3.   Transvesical (suprapubic), retropubic, transurethral, perineal.

4.   Hepatic and coeliac branches; nerves of Latarjet to pylorus and part of antrum.

5.   Numerous operations include supraradical, radical, simple, modified simple and sector mastectomies; wedge excision and 'lumpectomy'.

6.   Keller.

7.   Embolectomy using a Fogarty catheter.

8.   Pyloromyotomy.

9.   'Low' approach — below inguinal ligament; 'high' approach (Lotheissen) — through inguinal canal; McEvedy's approach — through rectus sheath; bilateral — through Pfannenstiel-type incision.

10.   Head and neck of pancreas, duodenum and pylorus, part of common bile duct.

11.   At operation, either by a choledochotomy or via a duodenal approach to the ampulla (usually combined with a sphincterotomy or sphincteroplasty). A 'missed' stone can be removed post-operatively with an instrument passed into the T-tube track, or using a duodenoscope and stone-snare passed through the ampulla.

12.   Extraserosal, that is not through the pleural or peritoneal cavities.

13.   Lienorenal ligament — apart from the abdominal wall!

14.   Anderson—Hynes pyeloplasty.

15.   Metastatic breast cancer, Cushing's syndrome, Conn's syndrome, phaeochromocytoma, adrenal virilism.

16.   Hind-quarter, above knee, through-knee, Gritti—Stokes, below knee, Symes, transmetatarsal toe amputations are examples.

17.   Carcinoma of bronchus, other primary tumours, solitary secondary tumours, bronchiectasis, lung abscess, pulmonary tuberculosis, are some indications.

18.   Cervical (supraclavicular), axillary (second rib space), posterior approach (bed of third rib).

19.   Lumbar 2 and 3.

20.   Numerous operations include Ivalon sponge rectopexy, rectosigmoidectomy, anterior resection, Thiersch wire.

1. *The following operations are performed on the stomach*:

(a) Billroth I
(b) Rammstedt
(c) Polya
(d) Devine exclusion
(e) Mayo

2. *The following described orthopaedic operations*:

(a) McBurney
(b) McMurray
(c) MacIntosh
(d) MacEwen
(e) MacTavish

3. *The following conditions are usually treated by total excision of the diseased organ*:

(a) Papillary carcinoma of thyroid

(b) Carcinoma of gastric antrum
(c) Carcinoma of kidney
(d) Hodgkin's disease
(e) Carcinoma of penis

4. *Surgery becomes necessary in most cases of*:

(a) Hiatus hernia
(b) Ulcerative colitis
(c) Thyrotoxicosis
(d) Carcinoma of prostate
(e) Otitis media

5. *Blood transfusion is commonly required in the following operations*:

(a) Aorto-iliac endartectomy
(b) Prostatectomy
(c) Cholecystectomy
(d) Abdominoperineal excision of rectum
(e) Mid-thigh amputation

Target scores U.G. 13, P.G. 19

1. (a)   T   Partial gastrectomy and gastroduodenostomy
   (b)   T   Pyloromyotomy for pyloric stenosis in infants
   (c)   T   Gastrectomy and gastrojejunostomy
   (d)   T   Rarely performed for inoperable antral carcinoma
   (e)   F   No gastric operation

2. (a)   F   He spent more time with the appendix!
   (b)   T   Osteotomy of femur
   (c)   T   Arthroplasty of knee
   (d)   T   Osteotomy of femur
   (e)   F

3. (a)   F   Hemithyroidectomy is usually curative, although some surgeons remove part of the other lobe
   (b)   F   Most antral carcinomas can be treated by subtotal gastrectomy
   (c)   T
   (d)   F   Radiotherapy or chemotherapy are primary treatments
   (e)   F   Radiotherapy or partial amputation are usually adequate

4. (a)   F   Medical treatment controls most cases
   (b)   F   Most cases settle without surgery
   (c)   F   Medical or ^{131}I treatments are satisfactory for many
   (d)   F   Hormone treatment is mainstay of therapy
   (e)   F   Antibiotics control vast majority

5. (a)   T
   (b)   T
   (c)   F
   (d)   T
   (e)   F

The following 16 physical signs and clinical tests are defined in three ways. Can you spot the correct definition?

(a)   *Boas' sign*:

1.   The demonstration of unilateral arm hypertension in a case of coarctation of the aorta.
2.   The demonstration of an area of hyperaesthesia in the scapula area in a case of acute cholecystitis.
3.   The demonstration of an area of dullness to percussion in the left upper quadrant in a case of splenic haematoma from trauma.

(b)   *Rovsing's sign*:

1.   The demonstration of bilateral renal swelling in a case of polycystic kidney.
2.   Attacks of flushing in patients with a carcinoid tumour.
3.   Right iliac fossa pain produced by palpation in the left iliac fossa in a case of appendicitis.

(c)   *Troisier's sign*:

1.   Discoloration of the umbilicus in a case of acute pancreatitis.
2.   The demonstration of an enlarged Virchow node in a patient with carcinoma of the stomach.
3.   Thrombophlebitis migrans.

(d)   *Kehr's sign*:

1.   Shoulder pain from blood under the diaphragm.
2.   An area of hyperaesthesia on the shoulder from subphrenic abscess.
3.   The passage of blood at the end of micturition in a case of Hunner's cystitis.

(e)   *Trousseau's sign*:

1.   In a case of tetany, tapping of the facial nerve produces twitching of the corner of the mouth.
2.   Spontaneous main d'accoucheur in a case of tetany.
3.   Fleeting migratory superficial thrombophlebitis.

(f)   *The sign of the Vas*:

1.   The looping down of the vas into the upper scrotum in a case of retractile testis. This is not found in a true undescended testis.
2.   The fact that the vas is usually normal in testicular tumours but often thickened in a case of epididymo-orchitis.
3.   The demonstration that the temporal artery becomes 'vas-like' when involved with temporal arteritis.

(g)   *Murphy's sign*:

1.   Subcostal tenderness on deep breathing.
2.   A subcostal mass on deep breathing.
3.   Subcostal rebound tenderness in a case of biliary colic.

(h)   *Angell's sign*:

1.   The dilating pupil on the side of an intracranial haemorrhage.
2.   The demonstration of rebound tenderness over an inflamed appendix.
3.   In a case of testicular torsion the opposite testis tends to lie horizontally in the standing position.

(i)   *McMurray's test*:

1.   Limitation of external rotation of the hip in a case of osteo-arthritis of the hip.
2.   Knee flexion and rotation to demonstrate a torn meniscus.
3.   The demonstration of increased lumbar lordosis in a patient lying flat when marked osteo-arthritis of both hips is present.

(j)   *Von Graefe's sign*:

1.   The absence of forehead wrinkling when a patient with exophthalmos looks up.
2.   Lid-lag in exophthalmos.
3.   Impaired corneal sensitivity in exophthalmos.

(k)   *Hippocratic facies*:

1.   The appearance of a patient with gross dehydration.
2.   The hectic flush and herpes labialis in a patient with lobar pneumonia.
3.   The appearance of a saddle nose and interstitial keratitis in a patient with congenital syphilis.

(l)   *The lavatory sign*:

1.   The demonstration of mucous diarrhoea due to a pelvic abscess, for example after appendicitis.
2.   Severe sudden chest pain when straining at stool in a case of pulmonary embolism after surgery.
3.   The presence of rectal pain in a case of ectopic pregnancy.

(m)   *Trendelenburg's sign*:

1.   The demonstration of saphenofemoral incompetence on coughing.
2.   The use of a tourniquet to demonstrate the site of perforating varicose veins.
3.   When a patient with congenital dislocation of the hip stands on the affected leg the pelvis tilts toward the opposite side.

(n)   *McBurney's sign*:

1.   One fingertip pressure over McBurney's point produces maximum tenderness in a case of appendicitis.
2.   The patient points to McBurney's point as the site of maximum pain in acute appendicitis.
3.   The demonstration of paraesthesia of the skin over McBurney's point in a case of acute appendicitis.

(o)   *Romberg's test*:

1.   Second urine sample passed becomes clear in a case of chronic prostatitis.
2.   Unsteadiness on standing with the eyes closed in a case of tabes dorsalis.
3.   Unilateral upgoing toe with contralateral pupil abnormality.

(p)   *Paget's test*:

1.   The fact that a cyst feels softer in the centre, and a solid harder at the centre.
2.   The demonstration of a temperature increase over a localised area with Paget's disease.
3.   The use of transillumination in the diagnosis of a hydrocoele.

Target scores U.G. 7, P.G. 10

(a)   *Boas' sign*

2.   Scapular area hyperaesthesia in acute cholecystitis.

(b)   *Rovsing's sign*

3.   Sign in appendicitis when palpation in the left iliac fossa produces pain in the right iliac fossa (probably due to caecal distension).

(c)   *Troisier's sign*

2.   The finding of a hard node in the left supraclavicular fossa in a patient with carcinoma of the stomach.

(d)   *Kehr's sign*

1.   Shoulder pain and hyperaesthesia from blood under the diaphragm, in ectopic pregnancy or ruptured spleen, for example.

(e)   *Trousseau's sign*

3.   Migratory superficial thrombophlebitis secondary to visceral carcinoma, of the pancreas, for example. (He demonstrated this sign on himself. His other sign is carpopedal spasm when a blood-pressure cuff is left inflated on the arm in hypocalcaemia.)

(f)   *The sign of the Vas*

2.   The vas is abnormal in epididymo-orchitis compared to testicular tumour.

(g)   *Murphy's sign*

1.   Right subcostal tenderness over an inflamed gall-bladder on deep breathing.

(h)   *Angell's sign*

3.   Demonstration of a horizontally lying testis on the opposite side to a suspected torsion. It is common to find a congenitally abnormal 'bell-clapper' testis in this condition.

(i)   *McMurray's test*

2.   Knee movements to demonstrate a torn meniscus.

(j)   *Von Graefe's sign*

2.   Demonstration of lid-lag in exophthalmos.

(k)   *Hippocratic facies*

1.   The signs of gross fluid and electrolyte loss, typically from peritonitis.

(l)   *The lavatory sign*

3.   Rectal pain in ruptured ectopic pregnancy.

(m)   *Trendelenburg's sign*

3.   The pelvic tilt of a patient with congenital hip dislocation standing on the affected leg.

(n)   *McBurney's sign*

1.   McBurney's point is the site of maximum tenderness in acute appendicitis.

(o)   *Romberg's test*

2.   Demonstration of unsteadiness in tabes when patient stands still with eyes closed.

(p)   *Paget's test*

1.   A cyst feels softer at the centre — a solid feels harder at the centre.

SECTION 2

Surgical mazes

SURGICAL MAZES

Try your skill at extricating yourself from these ten surgical mazes. You score according to the number of steps it takes to emerge from the maze. Par for the course is 100! (that is 10 steps for each maze). Start with No. 1 — if you think this statement is true, turn to 31; if you think it is false, turn to 47, and so on. Two wrong answers in a row will mean a backtrack.

		True	False
1.	Haemolytic disease predisposes to gall-stones.	31	47
2.	The commonest adrenal tumour is a hypernephroma.	117	40
3.	The treatment of pyonephrosis is usually nephrectomy.	64	122
4.	Colic is the commonest symptom in paralytic ileus.	91	65
5.	Portal hypertension is commonly due to cirrhosis.	137	173
6.	Ten per cent of patients with claudication eventually develop gangrene; more die from myocardial infarction.	179	159
7.	A definition of an empyema is a collection of pus in the pleural cavity.	157	166
8.	Homan's sign is usually positive in deep vein thrombosis.	249	246
9.	Scaphoid fractures tend to be comminuted.	247	244
10.	The worst examples of exophthalmos occur in the euthyroid state.	238	227

	True	False
11. WRONG. (Most is swallowed air unless it is a closed-loop obstruction, which is uncommon.) Cat-gut is derived from sheep's intestine.	135	42
12. WRONG. (But it is fairly common.) Krukenburg tumours are multiple adenomatous gastric polyps.	85	74
13. CORRECT. Toxic megacolon is due to stercoral ulceration of the bowel.	136	46
14. WRONG. (The deposits do not produce clinically enlarged lymph nodes.) Cervical rib is a common cause of Raynaud's disease.	103	123
15. WRONG. (Bleeding is the commonest symptom.) Go back to 122.		
16. WRONG. (This is a catch question — it is an exotoxin, not an endotoxin.) Go back to 3.		
17. WRONG. (It is the other way round.) Go back to 31.		
18. WRONG. (It often becomes negative.) Exomphalos is common in thyrotoxicosis.	63	43
19. WRONG. (This is true.) Go back to 65.		
20. WRONG. (Caput medusae is the name given to the dilated peri-umbilical veins of severe portal hypertension.) Go back to 113.		
21. CORRECT. Hirschsprung's disease and congenital megacolon are the same condition.	87	99
22. WRONG. (Bones are commoner.) Hyperhidrosis can occur in the stomach.	71	113
23. CORRECT. 90 per cent of perforated peptic ulcers occur in the duodenum.	31	84
24. WRONG. (It is. Hepatoma is commoner than cholangioma.) Dumping is a post-gastrectomy syndrome of bilious vomiting half an hour after meals.	72	43
25. CORRECT. Chronic venous ulcers can turn malignant.	33	144
26. WRONG. (It is; not hyperspadias.) Venous obstruction does not lead to limb gangrene.	105	90
27. CORRECT. Spinal fractures can cause paralytic ileus.	149	70

	True	False
28. CORRECT. Old patients with massive haematemesis should be treated conservatively for as long as possible.	174	108
29. WRONG. (Mumps can produce all of these.) Most thoracic aneurysms are syphilitic.	109	132
30. CORRECT. Para-umbilical hernias are commonest in infancy.	118	82
31. CORRECT. Carcinoma of the ascending and transverse colon is more common than descending and sigmoid.	101	119
32. WRONG. (Non-functioning adenomas are common at post mortem.) The commonest complication of thyroidectomy is hypoparathyroidism.	89	135
33. CORRECT. The commonest medical indication for circumcision is paraphimosis.	62	86
34. WRONG. (It is the commonest type of glioma.) Back to 98.		
35. CORRECT. Marfan's syndrome predisposes to dissecting aneurysm.	180	172
36. CORRECT. The majority of abscesses are best managed conservatively with antibiotics.	116	218
37. WRONG. (There is a high incidence of carcinoma of the stomach in patients with pernicious anaemia.) 80 per cent of patients with haematemesis have acute or chronic peptic ulceration.	110	163
38. WRONG. (Curling's ulcers is the name given to gastroduodenal stress ulceration after burns.) Back to 21.		
39. CORRECT. Varicocoele is slightly more common on the left than the right.	134	122
40. CORRECT. 60 per cent of lip cancers affect the lower lip.	138	113
41. CORRECT. Well done. You have now finished No. 4. Try No. 5.		
42. WRONG. (It is!) Back to 132.		
43. CORRECT. Well done. You have finished. Now try No. 2.		
44. CORRECT. Most patients with intestinal obstruction have visible peristalsis.	198	27

	True	False

45.   WRONG. (It is true.) Go back to 180.

46.   CORRECT. The opposite of hypospadias is epispadias. — 90 — 26

47.   WRONG. (It does.) Most fatal pulmonary
emboli come from iliac veins rather than calf veins. — 23 — 76

48.   WRONG. (The mortality is too high.
Direct attack on the varices, for example by
injection or ligation, is better.) Go back to 65.

49.   CORRECT. 25 per cent of clinical
stage 1 breast cancers have microscopic lymph
node deposits. — 21 — 14

50.   CORRECT. Well done. You are out again!
Now try No. 8.

51.   WRONG. (It is true, unlike all other
hernias.) Go back to 196.

52.   WRONG. (We would stop operating if
it were!) Go back to 213.

53.   WRONG. (It can.) Go back to 46.

54.   WRONG. (It is painful, much more so
than cellulitis.) Go back to 2.

55.   WRONG. (Most arise in the sympathetic
chain.) Go back to 119.

56.   CORRECT. Most pituitary tumours are
chromophobe adenomas. — 121 — 190

57.   WRONG. (Although the classical cause,
venous bleeding, is fairly common as well.) Go
back to 180.

58.   WRONG. (They are. Congenital diverticula are rare.) Go back to 13.

59.   WRONG. (Bladder outlet obstruction
is rare in the female.) Parotid calculi are more
common than submandibular. — 81 — 110

60.   WRONG. (It is a fairly benign tumour.)
The commonest form of parotitis is acute bacterial. — 202 — 161

61.   WRONG. (It is the commonest cause of
jaundice persisting for several weeks.) Pyloric
stenosis in neonates causes vomiting from birth. — 245 — 213

62.   WRONG. (It is phimosis.) Surgery is
indicated in most patients with renal hypertension. — 92 — 132

SURGICAL MAZES

	True	*False*
63. WRONG. (This is a catch question. It reads exomphalos, not exophthalmos!) Go back to 123.		
64. WRONG. (Antibiotics, removal of obstructing lesion, or nephrostomy, may save the kidney.) The endotoxin of tetanus acts on the motor cells of the central nervous system.	16	39
65. CORRECT. Jejunal diverticula do not cause symptoms.	169	98
66. WRONG. (It does. Some 20 per cent of cases with total colitis for more than ten years develop a carcinoma.) Go back to 31.		
67. WRONG. (It does. Even after surgery 50 per cent of cases relapse.) Patients after truncal vagotomy tend to be constipated due to small-bowel paralysis.	107	25
68. CORRECT. Mastectomy is essential to alter radically the survival in breast carcinoma.	133	167
69. CORRECT. Pernicious anaemia pre-disposes to carcinoma of the stomach.	137	37
70. WRONG. (They can.) Endarterectomy is the same as arterial disobliteration.	149	96
71. WRONG. (Hyperhidrosis is excessive sweating!) Go back to 40.		
72. WRONG. (Dumping is epigastric bloating, sweating and faintness after meals, but not vomiting.) Go back to 87.		
73. WRONG. Oral cholecystogram gives better concentration in the gall-bladder. Go back to 4.		
74. CORRECT. Another name for the Wilms' tumour is nephroblastoma.	46	127
75. WRONG. (It can.) Caput medusae occurs in neurofibromatosis.	20	142
76. WRONG. (They do.) You have got two wrong in a row, go back to 1.		
77. WRONG. (Acquired aneurysms are very rare.) The commonest cause of death in untreated coarctation of the aorta is renal failure.	112	30

	True	False

78.   WRONG. (They are rare under the age
of 40.) The best treatment of bleeding varices is
emergency portacaval shunt.   48   98

79.   CORRECT. The treatment of actinomycosis
is penicillin.   210   242

80.   WRONG. (It is true.) Go back to 6.

81.   WRONG. (Submandibular are much more
common.) Go back to 137.

82.   CORRECT. Mallory—Weiss syndrome is
haematemesis due to vomiting producing a mucosal
tear in the oesophagus.   41   126

83.   CORRECT. The commonest site for blood
spread in carcinoma of the breast is the lungs.   22   40

84.   WRONG. (It is true.) The recurrence rate of
femoral hernia is greater than that of inguinal.   17   119

85.   WRONG. (Krukenberg tumours are ovarian
tumours due to transcoelomic spread from the
stomach.) Go back to 13.

86.   CORRECT. In intestinal obstruction most
of the gaseous distension is due to bacterial decom-
position of intestinal contents.   11   135

87.   CORRECT. The Mantoux reaction becomes
positive in Crohn's disease.   18   43

88.   CORRECT. There is a statistically increased
risk of duodenal ulcer and stomach cancer in blood
groups A and O, respectively.   214   50

89.   WRONG. (It is bleeding.) Go back to 86.

90.   CORRECT. Well done. You have finished.
Try No. 3.

91.   WRONG. (Pain is usually absent.) The best
way to demonstrate gall-stones is by intravenous
cholangiography.   73   153

92.   WRONG. (Most cases of renal hypertension
are not surgically correctable, for example chronic
pyelonephritis.) Go back to 33.

93.   CORRECT. Cholecystitis can occur without
gall-stones.   28   178

SURGICAL MAZES

	True	False

94. WRONG. (Carcinoma of the tonsil has a bad prognosis.) The commonest causes of arterial emboli are atrial fibrillation and myocardial infarction. — 207, 160

95. WRONG. (With lobectomy most papillary carcinomas of the thyroid have a normal life expectancy.) Mucoviscidosis is an alternative name for fibrocystic disease of the pancreas. — 201, 228

96. WRONG. (It is.) Go back to 44.

97. WRONG. (Most cases are due to the vesico-ureteric reflux, and infection in childhood.) Heparin is normally found in the body. — 207, 146

98. CORRECT. Measurement of urinary steroids gives a good guide to prognosis in the patient with breast cancer. — 155, 167

99. WRONG. (They are the same.) Curling's ulcers are due to severe burns. — 123, 38

100. WRONG. (It is due to *Streptococcus*.) Go back to 56.

101. WRONG. (Sigmoid is the commonest site.) Ulcerative colitis predisposes to colonic carcinoma. — 119, 66

102. WRONG. (Males are much more common.) Go back to 40.

103. WRONG. (Cervical rib is an occasional cause of Raynaud's phenomena.) Go back to 21.

104. CORRECT. Mumps can cause pancreatitis, mastitis, thyroiditis and oophoritis. — 33, 29

105. WRONG. (It can, with severe iliac thrombosis.) Go back to 74.

106. WRONG. (Most fistulas are low ones.) Go back to 167.

107. WRONG. (Vagotomy tends to produce diarrhoea.) Go back to 122.

108. CORRECT. Well done. Now try No. 6.

109. WRONG. (This was true 50 years ago!) Go back to 33.

110. CORRECT. There is evidence that the pill increases the risk of breast cancer. — 139, 180

	True	False

111.   WRONG. (Femoral hernias have the highest incidence of strangulation due to the tight femoral ring and canal.) Go back to 25.

112.   WRONG. (It is cerebrovascular accidents.) Go back to 167.

113.   CORRECT. Scleroderma can cause dysphagia.   13   75

114.   WRONG. (Although the cause is unknown, there is a strong association.) Go back to 28.

115.   WRONG. (The mortality is due to the associated brain damage.) A furuncle is an infected sweat-gland tumour.   186   120

116.   WRONG. (It is still a surgical aphorism that pus must be let out!) Ischaemic leg pain is relieved by elevation and made worse on dependency.   152   196

117.   WRONG. (Hypernephroma is renal adeno-carcinoma.) Erysipelas is intensely painful.   83   54

118.   WRONG. (Para-umbilical hernias almost exclusively occur in adults. They are umbilical in children.) Stress ulcers occur in 20 per cent of severe burns.   41   156

119.   CORRECT. Murphy's sign is a potato-sized mass in acute cholecystitis.   125   21

120.   CORRECT. 50 per cent of anorectal atresias are associated with a fistula.   218   225

121.   CORRECT. Meckel's diverticula usually produce complications.   221   140

122.   CORRECT. Crohn's disease recurs in over 50 per cent of cases treated surgically.   25   67

123.   CORRECT. The commonest primary liver tumour is a hepatoma.   87   24

124.   WRONG. (It is a poorly differentiated carcinoma.) Most patients with carcinoma of the bladder eventually come to cystectomy.   187   196

125.   WRONG. (Murphy's sign is subcostal tenderness on deep inspiration.) Only 15 per cent of ganglioneuromas arise in the adrenal.   49   55

126.   WRONG. (It is.) Ten per cent of phaeo-chromocytomas are bilateral, ten per cent malignant and ten per cent extra-adrenal.   41   164

SURGICAL MAZES

	True	*False*
127. WRONG. (It is.) Phaeochromocytomas may produce hyperglycaemia.	90	53
128. WRONG. (This is true.) Phaeochromo- cytomas are commonest in the elderly.	219	79
129. WRONG. (This is true.) Most patients with Cushing's syndrome have adrenal hyperplasia.	120	191
130. CORRECT. Most patients with Cushing's syndrome have an enlarged pituitary fossa.	241	248
131. CORRECT. You have finished. Try the last maze, No. 10.		
132. CORRECT. Most adrenal adenomas are non-functioning.	86	32
133. WRONG. (Local excision of the carcinoma produces the same life expectancy, although this has a higher incidence of local recurrence.) Many fistulas in ano run above the levator ani muscle.	106	30
134. WRONG. (It is very rare on the right.) Most patients with carcinoma of the rectum have bleeding *per rectum*.	25	15
135. CORRECT. Well done. You have finished. Now try No. 4.		
136. WRONG. (Toxic megacolon occurs in severe ulcerative colitis and is liable to perforate.) The vast majority of bladder diverticula are due to bladder outlet obstruction.	74	58
137. CORRECT. 95 per cent of bladder diverticula occur in the male.	110	59
138. WRONG. (It is more like 90 per cent lower lip.) Bladder cancer is far more common in the male.	113	102
139. WRONG. (If anything, the contraceptive pill protects against breast cancer on present evidence.) Superficial burns are more painful than deep burns.	35	168
140. CORRECT. Well done! You have finished all 10. How did you score?		
141. WRONG. (It is true, even though a rare tumour.) Extradural haemorrhage is nearly always due to a middle meningeal haemorrhage.	57	93
142. CORRECT. In extradural haemorrhage there is nearly always a lucid interval.	12	13

	True	False
143. WRONG. (It is true.) 50 per cent of subdural haematomas are bilateral.	205	192
144. WRONG. (They can turn malignant and are then called Marjolin's ulcers.) The commonest hernia to strangulate is femoral.	104	111
145. WRONG. (It is true.) Go back to 93.		
146. WRONG. (Heparin is present in mast cells.) Go back to 179.		
147. WRONG. (Only a minority.) Go back to 88.		
148. WRONG. (It is nearer 90 per cent.) 80 per cent of patients with acute pancreatitis have gall-stones.	197	44
149. CORRECT. Well done. You have finished. Now try No. 7.		
150. WRONG. (It is true.) Go back to 158.		
151. WRONG. (It is only 50 per cent.) Go back to 120.		
152. WRONG. (Arterial ischaemia is better with dependency.) Go back to 218.		
153. CORRECT. Rodent ulcers usually start under the age of 40.	78	65
154. WRONG. (Radiotherapy has no place in the treatment of symptomless inoperable lung cancer.) Go back to 5.		
155. WRONG. (They are of little use in the individual case.) The commonest primary brain tumour is an astrocytoma.	68	34
156. WRONG. (Gastroduodenal haemorrhage is common in severe burns.) Go back to 82.		
157. WRONG. (The definition of an empyema is a collection of pus in a normal body cavity; it can also be found in the antrum and gall-bladder.) Gall-stones occur in 20 per cent of women over the age of 40 and in 20 per cent of men over the age of 70.	203	184
158. CORRECT. The mortality of acute pancreatitis is 10—15 per cent.	27	204

	True	False
159. WRONG. (It is true. One-third of claudicants improve, one-third stay the same, and a third will get worse, and of the latter another third develop gangrene.) The highest incidence of perforated peptic ulcer occurs between the ages of 45 and 55.	206	80
160. WRONG. It is true. Go back to 179.		
161. CORRECT. 20 per cent of head injuries develop intracranial haemorrhage.	233	56
162. WRONG. ('Gall-bladder dyspepsia' seems to be unrelated to gall-stones.) Go back to 27.		
163. WRONG. (It is true. Other causes for haematemesis are uncommon.) Go back to 137.		
164. WRONG. (These figures are correct.) Go back to 30.		
165. CORRECT. Killian's dehiscence occurs after abdominal wound breakdown.	235	176
166. CORRECT. Keloid scars are more common in children and coloured races.	120	129
167. CORRECT. 95 per cent of intracranial aneurysms are congenital.	82	77
168. WRONG. (Deep burns destroy the pain nerve endings.) Go back to 110.		
169. WRONG. (They can produce diverticulitis, bleeding and malabsorption.) Three-quarters of gastric ulcers will heal with medical treatment, but two-thirds of these will recur.	98	19
170. CORRECT. A subcapsular tear of the spleen must always be sutured.	200	210
171. CORRECT. Most lung cancers are un-differentiated.	131	193
172. WRONG. (It is true. Medionecrosis of the aorta may develop in this condition.) Half of the symptomless lung cancers are already inoperable.	93	45
173. WRONG. (It is true.) Radiotherapy is of no benefit in symptomless lung cancers.	69	154
174. WRONG. (Age is an indication for early surgery in bleeding ulcers.) Most gall-stones are asymptomatic.	108	145

	True	False

175.   WRONG. (It is true.) Go back to 165.
You are still almost home!

176.   CORRECT. Well done. Only two to go.
Try now No. 9.

177.   WRONG. (This is true.) Go back to 171.

178.   WRONG. (It can, although uncommonly.)
Sclerosing cholangitis is associated with ulcerative
colitis in 25 per cent of cases.   108   114

179.   CORRECT. Ureteric reflux is the
commonest cause of chronic pyelonephritis.   207   97

180.   CORRECT. Half the cases of sarcoma
of the prostate occur under the age of 5.   28   141

181.   WRONG. (It is true.) Go back to 10.

182.   CORRECT. Cystosarcoma phylloides
is a rare, very malignant tumour of the breast.   60   238

183.   WRONG. (This is true.) Go back to 161.

184.   WRONG. (These high statistics are correct.)
Go back to 7.

185.   WRONG. (This is true.) Go back to 238.

186.   WRONG. (A furuncle is a boil!) Go back
to 166.

187.   WRONG. (Most patients can be managed
with conservative treatment.) Go back to 218.

188.   WRONG. (It is a parotid tumour.) Go back
to 121.

189.   WRONG. (It is true.) Go back to 248.

190.   WRONG. (This is true.) Erysipelas is a
diffuse staphylococcal infection of the skin and
lymphatics.   100   201

191.   WRONG. (Hyperplasia is more common
than adenoma.) Go back to 166.

192.   WRONG. (It is true, unlike extradural
haematomas.) Go back to 207.

193.   WRONG. (They are.) The commonest
cause of epididymo-orchitis is mumps.   234   131

194.   WRONG. (There is a hazard of reaction
to antitetanus serum.) Patients with ulcerative
colitis treated by colectomy and ileostomy have
an increased risk of uric acid calculi.   131   177

	True	False
195. CORRECT. Papillary carcinoma of the thyroid has a good prognosis.	56	95
196. CORRECT. A carbuncle is a discharging abscess of the occipital muscles.	230	88
197. WRONG. (Too high. The figure is nearer 40—50 per cent.) Go back to 158.		
198. WRONG. (Most patients are too well covered to see it!) Cholecystectomy cures flatulent dyspepsia in gall-stone patients in only 50 per cent of cases.	149	162
199. WRONG. (Some testicular tumours can give rise to a positive pregnancy test.) Go back to 201.		
200. WRONG. (You do not suture it, you take it out!) Fracture of the head of the radius is one of the commonest fractures in the upper limb in young adults.	213	243
201. CORRECT. Colles' fracture is common in children.	231	121
202. WRONG. (It is mumps.) Go back to 238.		
203. CORRECT. The mortality of subdural haemorrhage is more than 50 per cent.	166	115
204. WRONG. (The overall mortality of acute pancreatitis is still high in spite of recent advances.) Ten per cent of the world's population is infected with *Entamoeba histolytica*.	44	150
205. CORRECT. 50 per cent of tumours of the oral cavity are squamous cell carcinomas.	148	158
206. CORRECT. Carcinoma of the tonsil is usually poorly differentiated.	179	94
207. CORRECT. Laryngeal papillomas are more common in children than in adults.	158	143
208. CORRECT. 95 per cent of carcinomas of the larynx are squamous cell carcinomas.	246	128
209. WRONG. (It is true.) Go back to 79.		
210. CORRECT. The commonest cause of prolonged jaundice in neonates is biliary atresia.	165	61
211. CORRECT. 40 per cent of neuro-blastomas arise in the adrenal.	244	239

	True	*False*

212.   WRONG. (It is a duct papilloma.)
Go back to 244.

213.   CORRECT. 60 per cent of inguinal
hernias occur on the right side, 20 per cent on
the left, and 20 per cent are bilateral.   165   232

214.   WRONG. (It is the other way round.)
Most umbilical hernias close spontaneously.   50   51

215.   WRONG. (Surgery is rarely necessary
in acute cholecystitis.) The prognosis of tetanus
is inversely proportional to the incubation
period.   161   185

216.   CORRECT. Polycystic kidney is
frequently familial.   248   229

217.   WRONG. (It is true.) Go back to 130.

218.   CORRECT. The commonest tumour
of the tonsil is a reticulosis.   124   88

219.   WRONG. (They are commonest in
young adults.) Go back to 246.

220.   WRONG. (There is a high incidence
of Down's syndrome in this condition.) In a
perforated duodenal ulcer plain X-rays show
air under the diaphragm in over 90 per cent
of cases.   236   237

221.   WRONG. (Most Meckel's are
asymptomatic.) Pregnancy tests can be
positive in men.   140   199

222.   WRONG. (This is true.) In intestinal
obstruction rebound tenderness implies
strangulation.   79   250

223.   WRONG. (It is true.) The commonest
cause of extrahepatic jaundice is carcinoma of
the pancreas.   240   130

224.   WRONG. (Mild cases do well with
medical treatment.) Go back to 9.

225.   WRONG. (It is true. Usually the urethra
or vagina.) 50 per cent of patients with carcinoma
of the head of the pancreas have a palpable gall-
bladder.   36   151

226.   WRONG. (Zollinger–Ellison syndrome
is much rarer than this.) Go back to 8.

	True	False

227. WRONG. (Progressive exophthalmos continues in spite of correction of thyroid function.) 90 per cent of mixed salivary tumours occur in the parotid. — 182 — 181

228. WRONG. (They are the same condition.) Go back to 56.

229. WRONG. (It is often familial.) Unilateral undescended testes are four times as common as bilateral. — 237 — 189

230. WRONG. (A carbuncle is a subcutaneous abscess usually on the back of the neck.) Most chest injuries require thoracotomy. — 147 — 50

231. WRONG. (A true Colles' fracture is rare in children.) Adenolymphoma is a rare primary lymph gland tumour. — 188 — 140

232. WRONG. (These statistics are correct.) Over half of thyroxine is iodine by molecular weight. — 176 — 175

233. WRONG. (This figure is too high.) In acute limb ischaemia muscle dies first, then nerves, then skin. — 195 — 183

234. WRONG. (This is a catch question. Mumps does not produce epididymitis — sorry.) Go back to 237.

235. WRONG. (This is the name for the weak area between the pharyngeal constrictors that produces a pharyngeal pouch.) The mortality of vagotomy and pyloroplasty is five per cent. — 52 — 176

236. WRONG. (Subdiaphragmatic air only occurs in 80 per cent.) Go back to 248.

237. CORRECT. Antitetanus serum should be given to every patient with a dirty wound. — 194 — 171

238. CORRECT. Acute cholecystitis usually subsides with medical treatment. — 161 — 215

239. WRONG. (It is true.) The commonest cause of bleeding from the nipple is carcinoma of the breast. — 212 — 130

240. WRONG. (Gall-stones are a more common cause.) Go back to 244.

241. WRONG. (Most do not.) Most oesophageal perforations are iatrogenic. — 216 — 217

	True	False

242.　　WRONG. (Penicillin is still the best drug for actinomycosis.) Half the cases of oesophageal atresia are associated with maternal hydramnios.　　170　　209

243.　　WRONG. (It is true if you do not count the clavicle as part of the upper limb!) Sorry, back to 210.

244.　　CORRECT. Cardiospasm is an alternative name for achalasia.　　130　　223

245.　　WRONG. (The vomiting does not commence for a week or so.) Go back to 210.

246.　　CORRECT. 80 per cent of patients with hypertrophic pyloric stenosis are male. 50 per cent are first-born.　　79　　222

247.　　WRONG. (A single, often hairline, fracture is usual.) Congenital hypertrophic pyloric stenosis should always be treated surgically.　　224　　211

248.　　CORRECT. There is an association between duodenal atresia and mongolism.　　171　　220

249.　　WRONG. (Homan's sign is only positive in a minority of cases of deep vein thrombosis.) Zollinger—Ellison's syndrome is the cause of peptic ulceration in three per cent of cases.　　226　　208

250.　　WRONG. (Rebound tenderness usually means local peritonitis.) Go back to 246.

SECTION 3

Differential diagnosis countdown

DIFFERENTIAL DIAGNOSIS COUNTDOWN

See how well you can score on causes of these common symptoms.

COUNTDOWN NO. 1

10 Causes of diarrhoea

9 Causes of anaemia

8 Causes of coma

7 Causes of enlarged lymph nodes

6 Causes of jaundice

5 Causes of haematemesis

4 Causes of abdominal distension

3 Causes of swelling of the leg

2 Causes of portal hypertension

1 Cause of pneumaturia

These lists give main causes and guides to classification. They are not intended to be exhaustive.

10 Causes of diarrhoea

Infective: for example *Salmonella, Shigella, Amoebae, Cholera.*

Malabsorption: chronic pancreatitis, obstructive jaundice, coeliac disease, blind-loop syndrome, mucoviscidosis, protein-losing enteropathy, etc.

Local bowel pathology: for example, ulcerative colitis, Crohn's disease, carcinoma of the colon, diverticular disease.

Hormonal: thyrotoxicosis, carcinoid syndrome, Zollinger—Ellison syndrome, etc.

Drugs: antibiotics, laxatives, for example.

9 Causes of anaemia

Iron deficiency: dietary; post-haemorrhagic, such as menorrhagia, peptic ulceration, carcinoma of the stomach, carcinoma of the rectum, parasites.

Megaloblastic: for example vitamin B_{12}, folate deficiency.

Haemolytic: examples are spherocytosis, haemoglobinopathies, haemolytic disease of new-born, auto-immune haemolytic anaemias.

Other causes: vitamin C deficiency (scurvy), myxoedema, bone marrow failure, chronic infection.

8 Causes of coma

CNS lesions: for example trauma, meningitis, encephalitis, subarachnoid haemorrhage, cerebrovascular accident, tumour — primary, secondary.

Metabolic: for example, diabetes, uraemia, liver failure.

Poisons: for example, barbiturate/salicylate/etc., overdose, carbon monoxide poisoning, alcohol.

7 Causes of enlarged lymph nodes

Infections: non-specific bacterial, specific (for example TB, syphilis, brucellosis), viral (for example glandular fever, rubella), fungal (for example blastomycosis), filariasis, etc.

Neoplastic: leukaemias, reticuloses (such as Hodgkin's disease), secondary carcinoma.

6 Causes of jaundice

Pre-hepatic: haemolytic anaemias such as spherocytosis.

Hepatic: congenital, for example Dubin—Johnson syndrome, infective (infective hepatitis, leptospirosis, liver abscess), toxic (poisons, such as carbon tetrachloride), drugs (halothane, chlorpromazine, for example).

Obstructive: gall-stones, carcinoma of the pancreas, carcinoma of the ampulla, duodenum, bile ducts.

5 Causes of haematemesis

Acute gastric erosions.

Duodenal ulceration.

Gastric ulceration.

Hiatus hernia.

Carcinoma of the stomach.

Mallory—Weiss syndrome.

Bleeding disorders.

Oesophageal varices.

4 Causes of abdominal distension

Fat.

Fluid: ascites (for example hepatic disease, peritoneal malignancy or inflammation), cyst (for example ovarian or pancreatic).

Flatus: intestinal obstruction (examples are carcinoma of the colon, adhesions, obstructed hernia).

Faeces: constipation.

Foetus: pregnancy.

3 Causes of swelling of the leg

Fluid retention: for example congestive cardiac failure, nephrotic syndrome.

Venous obstruction: such as deep vein thrombosis.

Lymphatic: for example congenital hypoplasia, blocked lymphatics — tumour, radiotherapy, filariasis.

2 Causes of portal hypertension

Cirrhosis: cardiac, nutritional, biliary.

Portal vein thrombosis: for example umbilical sepsis.

Budd—Chiari syndrome: hepatic vein obstruction, portal hepatitis.

1 Cause of pneumaturia

Vesicocolic fistula, for example diverticular disease, tumour, rarely cystitis with gas-forming organisms.

COUNTDOWN NO. 2

10 Causes of abdominal pain

9 Causes of hepatomegaly

8 Causes of haematuria

7 Causes of bleeding *per rectum*

6 Causes of a lump in the groin

5 Causes of shock

4 Causes of midline swelling in the anterior neck

3 Causes of a mass in the left iliac fossa

2 Causes of ascites

1 Cause of amino-aciduria

10 Causes of abdominal pain

Upper abdomen: peptic ulcer, gall-stones, pancreatic pain (pancreatitis for example), renal pain (such as hydronephrosis), hepatic pain (hepatitis or tumour, for example).

Mid-abdomen: small-gut colic (adhesions, obstruction, for example).

Lower abdomen: ureteric colic, appendicitis, carcinoma of the colon, diverticular disease, gynaecological (salpingitis for example), cystitis, carcinoma of the bladder.

9 Causes of hepatomegaly

Infective: examples are infectious hepatitis, liver abscess, amoebic hepatitis, hydatid disease.

Cirrhosis: such as cardiac, Laennec's, biliary.

Infiltrations: for example fatty degeneration, lipid steroid diseases, amyloid, haemochromotosis.

Tumours: primary, such as hepatoma, secondary, as gastric carcinoma.

8 Causes of haematuria

General: bleeding disorders.

Upper tract: trauma, infection, calculi, acute and chronic nephritis, hydronephrosis, polycystic disease, tumour.

Lower tract: cystitis, carcinoma of the bladder, prostatic hypertrophy, carcinoma of the prostate, trauma.

7 Causes of bleeding per rectum

Anal: for example haemorrhoids, fissure, fistula, tumour.

Rectal: proctitis, ulcerative colitis, carcinoma, adenoma, etc.

Colonic: examples are colitis, carcinoma, polyps, diverticulitis.

Upper tract: bleeding duodenal ulcer, Meckel's diverticulum, for example.

6 Causes of a lump in the groin

Hernia: inguinal, femoral, for example.

Lymph gland: for example inflammation, tumour — primary and secondary.

Vascular: saphena varix, aneurysm, etc.

Miscellaneous: lipoma, maldescended testis, hydrocoele of cord.

5 Causes of shock

Neurogenic: faint.

Hypovolaemic: bleeding, burns, fluid loss.

Cardiogenic: pulmonary embolism, acute heart failure, myocardial infarction.

Septicaemia.

Anaphylactic.

4 Causes of raised intracranial pressure

Hydrocephalus.

Trauma: cerebral oedema, haematoma.

Abscess, meningitis, encephalitis.

Tumours: primary, secondary.

3 Causes of a mass in the left iliac fossa

Examples are:

Ovarian — cyst, tumour.

Colonic — diverticular disease, tumour.

Uterine — fibroid.

Urinary — pelvic kidney, carcinoma ureter or bladder.

2 Causes of ascites

Cirrhosis, portal hypertension.

Peritoneal inflammation or malignancy.

Congestive cardiac failure.

Nephrotic syndrome.

1 Cause of amino-aciduria

Fanconi syndrome.

Cystinuria.

Phenylketonuria.

COUNTDOWN NO. 3

10 Causes of back pain

9 Causes of weight loss

8 Causes of painful shoulder

7 Causes of pain in the chest

6 Causes of leg ulceration

5 Causes of pain in the testes

4 Causes of a rectoperitoneal mass

3 Causes of neonatal intestinal obstruction

2 Causes of dark brown urine — not due to blood

1 Cause of pigmentation in the mouth

10 Causes of back pain

Trauma/degenerative: for example acute back strain, oesteo-arthrosis, prolapsed disc, spondylolisthesis, scoliosis.

Inflammatory: rheumatoid arthritis, ankylosing spondylitis.

Metabolic: osteomalacia, osteoporosis, hyperparathyroidism, for example.

Neoplastic: for example secondary deposits, primary tumour — Hodgkin's, myeloma.

Vascular: aortic aneurysm, for example.

Renal: hydronephrosis, carcinoma, calculi, for example.

Referred pain: for example salpingitis, pancreatitis.

9 Causes of weight loss

Gastro-intestinal disease: examples are peptic ulceration, cirrhosis, malabsorption as in pancreatitis and gluten enteropathy.

Metabolic: thyrotoxicosis, diabetes, Addison's disease, uraemia, etc.

Malignant disease: for example carcinoma of the bronchus, gastro-intestinal malignancy, hepatic malignancy.

Chronic infections: TB for example.

Dietary restriction.

8 Causes of painful shoulder

Local disease or trauma: such as dislocation, arthropathy (osteo-arthritis, rheumatoid and septic arthritis), subacromial bursitis, supraspinatus tendinitis, tumours.

Referred pain: such as cholecystitis, diaphragmatic irritation (blood, perforation, sub-phrenic abscess).

7 Causes of pain in the chest

Chest wall: for example herpes, rib fracture, primary and secondary tumour, Bornholm disease.

Cardiac: myocardial infarction, angina pectoris, pericarditis, for example.

Vascular: for example pulmonary embolism, dissecting aneurysm.

Lung/pleura: examples are pneumonia, pleurisy, pneumothorax, primary and secondary tumours.

Oesophageal: reflux, diffuse oesophageal spasm.

6 Causes of leg ulceration

Gravitational: venous ulcer.

Ischaemic: atherosclerosis.

Traumatic: injury/burns.

Neurogenic: leprosy, for example.

Diabetic.

Blood dyscrasia: for example leukaemia, haemolytic anaemia.

Infective: examples are syphilis, TB, yaws, tropical ulcer.

5 Causes of pain in the testes

Inflammatory: such as epididymo-orchitis — non-specific or tuberculous.

Torsion: testis or appendages.

Tumours: seminoma or teratoma.

Hydrocoele, or cyst of epididymis.

Trauma.

Referred: ureteric colic.

4 Causes of a retroperitoneal mass

Renal: examples are hydronephrosis, cysts, tumour.

Pancreatic: such as cysts, tumour.

Lymph nodes: primary tumour, secondary tumour.

Vascular: aneurysm, for example.

Lipoma.

Liposarcoma, etc.

3 Causes of neonatal intestinal obstruction

Stenosis or atresia: duodenal, jejunal, ileum.

Anorectal agenesis.

Meconium ileum.

Volvulus neonatorum.

Congenital bands — associated malrotation.

Hirschsprung's disease

2 Causes of dark brown urine

Methaemoglobin — congenital methaemoglobinaemia.

Melanuria: for example secondary deposits of malignant melanoma.

Alkaptonuria.

Phenolic drugs.

1 Cause of pigmentation in the mouth

Addison's disease.

Arsenic bismuth silver toxicity.

Peutz—Jegher's syndrome.

COUNTDOWN NO. 4

10 Causes of arthropathy

9 Causes of albuminuria

8 Causes of haemoptysis

7 Causes of vomiting

6 Causes of facial palsy

5 Causes of a lump in the breast

4 Causes of a raised intracranial pressure

3 Causes of Raynaud's phenomena

2 Causes of arterial embolism

1 Cause of macroglossia

10 Causes of arthropathy

Congenital: such as achondroplasia, osteogenesis imperfecta.

Degenerative: such as osteo-arthritis.

Haematogenous: for example bleeding disorders such as haemophilia.

Infective: for example septic arthritis, gonococcus, TB.

Metabolic: amyloid, gout, osteomalacia, etc.

Vascular: for example polyarteritis nodosa, giant-cell arteritis.

Neoplastic: primary or secondary tumours.

Neuropathic: Charcot joints, for example.

Miscellaneous: ankylosing spondylitis, rheumatoid arthritis, sarcoidosis, are examples.

9 Causes of albuminuria

(A) Disease of urinary tract

Renal: acute and chronic glomerulonephritis, acute and chronic pyelonephritis, acute tubular necrosis, renal tuberculosis, renal tumour (Wilms' adenocarcinoma), calculi, hydronephrosis, polycystic disease.

Lower tract: tumour, infection, for example.

(B) Secondary albuminuria

Congestive failure.

Hypertension.

Toxaemia of pregnancy.

Amyloidosis.

Purpuras.

Myeloma.

8 Causes of haemoptysis

Upper respiratory tract: for example epistaxis, bleeding gums, carcinoma of the larynx.

Pulmonary disease: such as bronchitis, pneumonia, TB, carcinoma of the bronchus, secondary tumour, adenoma, trauma, pulmonary embolism.

215

DIFFERENTIAL DIAGNOSIS COUNTDOWN

7 Causes of vomiting

Central

Metabolic: such as uraemia, diabetes, hypercalcaemia.

Miscellaneous: such as pregnancy, psychogenic, raised intracranial pressure, drugs, Ménière's disease, labyrinthitis.

Gastro-intestinal: for example gastritis, peptic ulceration, carcinoma of the stomach, carcinoma of the pancreas, intestinal obstruction, peritonitis, appendicitis, biliary colic.

6 Causes of facial palsy

Upper motor neuron lesion: cerebrovascular accident, primary neoplasms, secondary neoplasms, trauma.

Lower motor neuron lesion: Bell's palsy, trauma, acoustic neuroma, meningitis, polyneuritis, parotid carcinoma, parotidectomy.

5 Causes of a lump in the breast

Cyst.

Chronic mastitis.

Fibro-adenoma (soft, hard, giant).

Duct papilloma.

Abscess.

Carcinoma.

4 Causes of a raised intracranial pressure

Hydrocephalus.

Meningitis.

Encephalitis.

Space-occupying lesion: for example haemorrhage (extradural, subdural, intra-cerebral, subarachnoid, intraventricular), abscess, tumour (primary and secondary).

3 Causes of Raynaud's phenomenon

Cervical rib.

Micro embolism — subclavian aneurysm.

Cold agglutination.

Systemic lupus erythematosis.

Ergot.

Buerger's disease.

Scleroderma.

2 Causes of arterial embolism

Cardiac: atrial fibrillation (for example rheumatic heart disease), myocardial infarction.

Arterial: thrombosis, atheromatous plaques.

1 Cause of macroglossia

Acromegaly.

Primary amyloidosis.

Cretinism.

Myxoedema.

COUNTDOWN NO. 5

10 Causes of dysphagia

9 Causes of renal enlargement

8 Causes of convulsions

7 Causes of swelling in the scrotum

6 Causes of an upper abdominal mass

5 Causes of anuria

4 Causes of a swelling in the parotid region

3 Causes of generalised lymphadenopathy

2 Causes of pneumoperitoneum

1 Cause of a urinary leak from the umbilicus

10 Causes of dysphagia

Lumen: foreign bodies.

Wall: inflammation (tonsillitis/pharyngitis; oesophagitis — reflux, corrosive, infection such as *Monilia*), pharyngeal pouch, diverticula oesophagus, achalasia, diffuse oesophageal spasm, scleroderma, tumours such as leiomyoma, carcinoma.

Outside: compression from aneurysm, goitre, glands, etc., involvement carcinoma of the bronchus.

Neurological: bulbar palsy, syringomyelia.

9 Causes of renal enlargement

Hypertrophy: such as absent other kidney.

Cysts: polycystic disease.

Infection: pyelonephritis, pyonephrosis, perinephric abscess, TB.

Trauma: haematoma.

Hydronephrosis: congenital, stones, tumours, bladder outlet obstruction.

Tumours: primary (Wilms', Grawitz, papillary), secondary.

8 Causes of convulsions

Idiopathic epilepsy.

Congenital: hydrocephalus, angioma.

Trauma.

Local infection: for example meningitis, encephalitis, abscess, cerebral malaria.

General infections: such as gastro-enteritis in infancy, febrile convulsions.

Metabolic: uraemia, hypoglycaemia, etc.

Cerebrovascular accidents.

Tumours: primary and secondary.

7 Causes of a swelling in the scrotum

'Cystic': hydrocoele, haematocoele, hernia, cyst of epididymis, spermatocoele, varicocoele.

Solid: epididymo-orchitis, torsion, tumour (seminoma, teratoma), gumma.

6 Causes of an upper abdominal mass

Hepatic: examples cirrhosis, tumour.

Gall bladder: for example mucocele.

Spleen: examples are spherocytosis, portal hypertension.

Stomach: carcinoma of the stomach, for example.

Pancreas: pseudocyst, for example.

Kidney: hydronephrosis, for example.

Transverse colon: for example carcinoma of the colon.

Vascular: aneurysm, for example.

5 Causes of anuria

Obstruction: calculus (solitary kidney), carcinoma of bladder or uterus involving ureter, retroperitoneal fibrosis.

Renal disease: acute tubular necrosis, chronic nephritis, chronic pyelonephritis, polycystic kidney, Crush syndrome, mismatched transfusion, malignant hypertension.

4 Causes of a swelling in the parotid region

Mumps.

Acute parotitis.

Mixed parotid tumour.

Calculus.

Foreign-body duct.

Sialectasis.

Carcinoma of parotid.

Adenolymphoma.

Sjögren's syndrome.

Enlargements of lymph nodes.

3 Causes of generalised lymphadenopathy

Leukaemias.

Reticuloses: Hodgkin's, lymphosarcoma, reticulum cell sarcoma.

Glandular fever.

Amyloidosis.

Sarcoidosis.

Systemic lupus erythematosis.

2 Causes of pneumoperitoneum

Trauma: stab wounds, operations, ruptured viscus.

Perforation viscus: perforated duodenal ulcer, diverticular disease, appendicitis.

1 Cause of a urinary leak from the umbilicus

Patent urachus.

Carcinoma of the bladder.

COUNTDOWN NO. 6

10 Causes of swelling of a bone

 9 Injuries caused by a fall on the outstretched hand

 8 Causes of an abnormal mediastinal shadow on chest X-ray

 7 Causes of a headache

 6 Causes of an enlarged thyroid

 5 Causes of splenomegaly

 4 Causes of gynaecomastia

 3 Causes of anal pain

 2 Causes of referred pain to the shoulder

 1 Cause of calcification in the liver

10 Causes of swelling of a bone

Traumatic: for example subperiosteal haematoma, fracture, callus.

Infective: such as osteomyelitis.

Metabolic: rickets, scurvy, acromegaly, osteitis fibrosa cystica, etc.

Paget's disease.

Tumours: such as osteoma, chondroma, osteoclastoma, osteosarcoma, Ewing's tumour, myeloma, secondary tumour.

9 Injuries caused by a fall on the outstretched hand

Fracture lower end of radius.

Fracture—separation lower radial epiphysis.

Fracture head or neck of radius.

Dislocation of elbow.

Supracondylar fracture.

Fracture—separation upper humeral epiphysis.

Fracture of clavicle.

Fracture of scaphoid.

Fracture shaft radius/ulnar.

Dislocation of shoulder.

Fracture neck of humerus.

8 Causes of an abnormal mediastinal shadow on chest X-ray

Lymph nodes: carcinoma of bronchus, reticulosis, sarcoidosis, secondary tumour such as carcinoma of oesophagus.

Oesophageal: achalasia, tumours, para-oesophageal hiatus hernia.

Cardiovascular: rheumatic heart disease, ventricular aneurysm, aortic aneurysm.

Thymus: thymoma.

Retrosternal goitre.

Skeletal: ganglioneuroma, bone tumours.

DIFFERENTIAL DIAGNOSIS COUNTDOWN

7 Causes of a headache

Intracranial lesion: such as trauma, tumour, cerebrovascular accident, aneurysm, meningitis, encephalitis.

Cranial: skull tumour, Paget's disease, for example.

Cervical spine: cervical spondylosis, rheumatoid arthritis, etc.

Eye: for example iritis, glaucoma.

ENT: sinusitis, middle-ear disease, for example.

General: drugs, uraemia, infection, hypertension, migraine, psychogenic, temporal arteritis.

6 Causes of an enlarged thyroid

Iodine-deficiency goitre: diffuse, multinodular.

Thyrotoxicosis.

Dishormonogenetic goitre.

Adenoma.

Thryoiditis: De Quervain's, auto-immune.

Carcinoma: papillary, follicular, medullary, anaplastic.

5 Causes of splenomegaly

Infective: for example malaria, glandular fever, Kala azar.

Haematological: polycythaemia, spherocytosis, leukaemia, idiopathic thrombo-cytopenic purpura, for example.

Reticuloses.

Portal hypertension.

Connective tissue disease: for example systemic lupus erythematosis, polyarteritis nodosa.

4 Causes of gynaecomastia

Drugs: for example oestrogen for carcinoma of the prostate, digoxin.

Cirrhosis.

Testicular tumours: for example interstitial cell tumour or teratoma.

Leprosy.

Orchidectomy.

Intersex states: for example Klinefelter's syndrome.

3 Causes of anal pain

Fissure.

Haemorrhoids (thrombosed or acute prolapse).

Fistula.

Abscess.

Carcinoma.

Proctalgia fugax.

2 Causes of referred pain to the shoulder

Gall-bladder disease: acute cholecystitis, biliary colic.

Pancreatic disease: pancreatitis.

Diaphragmatic irritation: subphrenic blood, abscess, perforated duodenal ulcer.

1 Cause of calcification in the liver

Hydatid.

Primary and secondary tumour.

Liver abscess

SECTION 4

The acute abdomen—case histories A to Z

Test your clinical acumen on these 26 case
histories. Starting with the presenting complaint
select the clinical features that you think are
important counting one point for each page you turn to.
Deduct the total from 25 to get your final score.

Case	U.G.	P.G.	Case	U.G.	P.G.
A	15	18	N	15	17
B	13	16	O	14	16
C	16	19	P	13	15
D	15	18	Q	14	16
E	14	17	R	10	13
F	18	20	S	10	13
G	11	13	T	12	14
H	12	14	U	13	15
I	10	12	V	10	12
J	11	14	W	10	12
K	10	12	X	11	13
L	13	15	Y	12	14
M	14	16	Z	12	14

CASE A.   Female, aged 55, married with 3 children, complaining of abdominal pain for 30 hours.

CASE B.   Female, aged 16, single secretary, complaining of 2 days of abdominal pain and weakness for 2 hours.

CASE C.   Male, aged 45, labourer, complaining of abdominal pain for 4 hours.

CASE D.   Female, aged 63, complaining of abdominal pain for 30 hours.

CASE E.   Female, aged 24, single, complaining of abdominal pain for 3 days.

CASE F.   Male, aged 15, schoolboy, complaining of abdominal pain for 20 hours.

CASE G.   Female, aged 35, complaining of abdominal pain and vomiting for 3 hours.

CASE H.   Female, aged 24, complaining of abdominal pain for 6 hours.

CASE I.   Female, aged 76, complaining of abdominal pain for 6 hours.

CASE J.   Baby, aged 6 months, screaming intermittently for 3 hours.

CASE K.   Two-day-old girl vomiting.

CASE L.   Female, aged 44, married housewife, complaining of abdominal pain for 3 hours.

CASE M.   Male, aged 60, driver involved in road accident, complaining of abdominal pain since accident.

CASE N.   Male, aged 38, steel erector, complaining of abdominal pain for 6 hours.

CASE O.   Female, aged 62, housewife, complaining of abdominal pain for 2 days.

CASE P.   Male, aged 30, draughtsman, complaining of abdominal pain and diarrhoea for 3 days.

CASE Q.   Girl, aged 9, complaining of abdominal pain for 6 hours.

CASE R.   Female, aged 54, housewife, complaining of abdominal pain for 10 hours.

CASE S.   Two-day-old neonate, male, vomiting since birth.

CASE T.   Female, aged 81, complaining of abdominal pain for 10 hours.

CASE U.   Female, aged 13, with a history of 4 hours of abdominal pain.

CASE V.   Female, aged 32, complaining of abdominal pain for 12 hours.

CASE W.   Female, aged 65, complaining of abdominal pain for 6 hours.

CASE X.   Male, aged 72, retired sailor, complaining of abdominal pain for 2 hours.

CASE Y.   Male, aged 68, retired, complaining of abdominal pain for 6 hours.

CASE Z.   Female, aged 47, 3 children, complaining of abdominal pain for 4½ hours.

CASE A.   Right upper quadrant.

CASE B.   Right iliac fossa and hypogastrium.

CASE C.   Epigastrium and right iliac fossa.

CASE D.   Left iliac fossa and hypogastrium.

CASE E.   Right iliac fossa and hypogastrium.

CASE F.   Central, then moving to right iliac fossa.

CASE G.   Central.

CASE H.   Hypogastric.

CASE I.   Generalised.

CASE J.   Unknown.

CASE K.   None.

CASE L.   Epigastrium.

CASE M.   Generalised and left chest.

Other features on pages:

CASE N.   Left flank and left iliac fossa.

CASE O.   Hypogastric.

CASE P.   Central and left iliac fossa.

CASE Q.   Right iliac fossa and hypogastrium.

CASE R.   Central.

CASE S.   None.

CASE T.   Central and generalised.

CASE U.   Right iliac fossa.

CASE V.   Right upper quadrant.

CASE W.   Left upper quadrant becoming generalised.

CASE X.   Generalised.

CASE Y.   Generalised.

CASE Z.   Hypogastric and left iliac fossa.

CASE A.   Right scapula.

CASE B.   Right shoulder.

CASE C.   Some shoulder pain.

CASE D.   None.

CASE E.   No radiation.

CASE F.   None.

CASE G.   None.

CASE H.   None.

CASE I.   None.

CASE J.   Unknown.

CASE K.   None.

CASE L.   Pain radiates to centre of back level T12.

CASE M.   Left shoulder.

Other features on pages:

CASE N.   Left loin and left testis.

CASE O.   None.

CASE P.   None.

CASE Q.   None.

CASE R.   None.

CASE S.   None.

CASE T.   None.

CASE U.   None.

CASE V.   Some radiation right posterior chest.

CASE W.   None.

CASE X.   Radiates to low back.

CASE Y.   None.

CASE Z.   None.

CASE A.   Pain constant and increasing but not severe. No colic.

CASE B.   Nagging ache in the right iliac fossa for 2 days, associated with some occasional colic. Pain is now generalised.

CASE C.   Sudden onset of severe pain which is constant. Pain has now become easier but more widespread.

CASE D.   Nagging constant ache.

CASE E.   Continuous nagging pain gradually increasing.

CASE F.   Some colic at first, now continuous dull ache.

CASE G.   Severe colic every 5 minutes.

CASE H.   Colic every 15 minutes. Fairly mild, some tenesmus.

CASE I.   Moderately severe colic.

CASE J.   Colic every 5 minutes with pain-free interval between.

CASE K.   None.

CASE L.   Sudden onset of severe constant pain.

CASE M.   Constant pain, not severe, but hurts to breathe.

CASE N.　　　Severe colic.

CASE O.　　　Dull colic every 15 minutes.

CASE P.　　　Moderately severe colic.

CASE Q.　　　Continuous nagging pain gradually increasing with occasional colic.

CASE R.　　　Moderately severe colic every few minutes.

CASE S.　　　None.

CASE T.　　　Colic every 15 minutes.

CASE U.　　　Constant ache.

CASE V.　　　Continuous severe pain.

CASE W.　　　Sudden onset, gradually increasing pain, not colicky.

CASE X.　　　Sudden onset, central abdominal pain, becoming generalised, still severe.

CASE Y.　　　Sudden onset, severe pain, starting in the left iliac fossa but now becoming generalised.

CASE Z.　　　Sudden onset of constant pain which is gradually increasing.

Other features on pages:

CASE A.   Very nauseated, vomited 3 times.

CASE B.   None.

CASE C.   Vomited once, now no nausea.

CASE D.   Nauseated, but not vomited.

CASE E.   Nauseated but no vomiting.

CASE F.   Nauseated, vomited once.

CASE G.   Has vomited 7 times, starting a few minutes after onset of abdominal colic.

CASE H.   Vomited 3 times at outset.

CASE I.   Vomited once.

CASE J.   Vomited once.

CASE K.   Vomited 6 times. Vomiting started 16 hours after birth.

CASE L.   Vomited 3 times.

CASE M.   None.

CASE N.   Vomited 4 times.

CASE O.   Nauseated, no vomiting.

CASE P.   None.

CASE Q.   Nauseated, and has vomited 4 times.

CASE R.   Vomited 5 times in the last 6 hours.

CASE S.   Vomited 6 times, vomiting not projectile.

CASE T.   Nauseated, and has vomited 3 times.

CASE U.   Slight nausea.

CASE V.   Vomited 3 times.

CASE W.   Nauseated but no vomiting.

CASE X.   Nauseated and has vomited once.

CASE Y.   Has vomited twice and is nauseated.

CASE Z.   Nauseated and has vomited once.

Other features on pages:

CASE A.   Anorexic. Weight 16 stone.

CASE B.   Normal. Weight steady.

CASE C.   Appetite good. Weight steady.

CASE D.   Anorexic. Weight steady at 8 stone.

CASE E.   Slight anorexia. Weight steady.

CASE F.   Anorexic 24 hours. Weight steady.

CASE G.   Appetite and weight previously good.

CASE H.   Normal until 6 hours ago.

CASE I.   Normal.

CASE J.   Taking feeds.

CASE K.   Not taking feeds.

CASE L.   Weight steady 11 stones. Anorexic since pain.

CASE M.   Appetite good. Weight steady.

CASE N.　　　　Normal.

CASE O.　　　　Anorexia for 2 days. Weight loss 1 stone in last 6 months.

CASE P.　　　　Appetite good. Weight loss 1 stone over 1 year.

CASE Q.　　　　Slight anorexia. Weight 6½ stone.

CASE R.　　　　No anorexia until last 10 hours. Weight 14 stone.

CASE S.　　　　Taking feeds satisfactorily but vomits immediately after feed.

CASE T.　　　　Anorexic 24 hours. Weight constant, 7 stone.

CASE U.　　　　No anorexia. Weight steady, 8 stone.

CASE V.　　　　Appetite good. Weight constant.

CASE W.　　　　Appetite normal until onset of pain. Weight steady.

CASE X.　　　　Slight recent weight loss.

CASE Y.　　　　Appetite and weight steady until onset of pain.

CASE Z.　　　　Slightly overweight.

Other features on pages:

CASE A.   Slightly constipated.

CASE B.   Regular.

CASE C.   Regular.

CASE D.   Diarrhoea for 2 days with some bleeding, dark red.

CASE E.   Regular.

CASE F.   Constipated for 2 days.

CASE G.   Bowels regular, passing flatus.

CASE H.   Diarrhoea 6 times, watery brown without any bleeding.

CASE I.   Bowels open regularly until yesterday; has not passed flatus for
            6 hours.

CASE J.   Little blood in nappy.

CASE K.   Has passed a little meconium.

CASE L.   Regular.

CASE M.   Bowels open regularly.

CASE N.   Normal.

CASE O.   Constipated for 3 days; some diarrhoea over the last 3 months. Is passing flatus.

CASE P.   Diarrhoea for 2 days, 6 times per day with blood and mucus.

CASE Q.   Regular.

CASE R.   Bowels open, has not passed flatus for 3 hours.

CASE S.   No meconium passed.

CASE T.   Constipated 30 hours, no flatus passed for the last 12 hours.

CASE U.   Regular.

CASE V.   Regular.

CASE W.   Slight diarrhoea with a little dark blood 3 hours ago.

CASE X.   Regular.

CASE Y.   Occasional diarrhoea, some bleeding *per rectum* a few months ago. Bowels have been regular for the last week.

CASE Z.   Regular.

CASE A. Normal.

CASE B. Normal.

CASE C. Normal.

CASE D. Frequency and dysuria.

CASE E. Some frequency and dysuria.

CASE F. Slight frequency.

CASE G. Normal.

CASE H. Normal.

CASE I. Normal.

CASE J. Normal.

CASE K. Normal.

CASE L. Normal.

CASE M. Normal.

CASE N.   Slight frequency and dysuria.

CASE O.   Normal.

CASE P.   Normal.

CASE Q.   Normal.

CASE R.   Normal.

CASE S.   Normal.

CASE T.   Normal.

CASE U.   Normal.

CASE V.   No symptoms but urine dark.

CASE W.   Normal.

CASE X.   Some prostatism.

CASE Y.   Normal.

CASE Z.   Slight frequency and dysuria.

CASE A.   Periods regular.

CASE B.   Last period 6 days late, previously regular.

CASE C.   Nil relevant.

CASE D.   Nil relevant.

CASE E.   Vaginal discharge, periods regular. Has just started last period.

CASE F.   Nil relevant.

CASE G.   Nil relevant.

CASE H.   Normal.

CASE I.   Nil relevant.

CASE J.   Nil relevant.

CASE K.   Nil relevant.

CASE L.   Nil relevant.

CASE M.   Nil relevant.

CASE N.   Nil relevant.

CASE O.   Short of breath on exercise for the last week.

CASE P.   Nil relevant.

CASE Q.   Has had a sore throat for 12 hours.

CASE R.   Periods stopped 12 months ago.

CASE S.   Is said to have a congenital murmur.

CASE T.   Nil relevant.

CASE U.   Last menstrual period 14 days ago, periods regular.

CASE V.   Husband says she is slightly jaundiced.

CASE W.   Short of breath, some ankle swelling.

CASE X.   Nil relevant.

CASE Y.   Smokes 25 cigarettes a day, chronic bronchitic, short of breath on one flight of stairs.

CASE Z.   Menopause 18 months ago.

CASE A.   Indigestion for many years.

CASE B.   Had salpingitis aged 15.

CASE C.   Indigestion for 7 years.

CASE D.   Nagging pain left iliac fossa for 3 years.

CASE E.   Appendicectomy aged 10.

CASE F.   Similar pain one year ago.

CASE G.   Partial gastrectomy for gastric ulcer one year ago.

CASE H.   Nil relevant.

CASE I.   Schizophrenic.

CASE J.   Nil relevant.

CASE K.   Nil relevant.

CASE L.   Gall-stones diagnosed 3 years ago. No operation. Well on fat-free diet.

CASE M.   Gastrectomy for duodenal ulcer 2 years ago.

CASE N.   Nil relevant.

CASE O.   Ovarian cyst removed 5 years ago (benign).

CASE P.   Similar episode 1 year ago. Has never been to the tropics.

CASE Q.   Appendicectomy aged 7.

CASE R.   Acute cholecystitis 2 months ago.

CASE S.   Mongol.

CASE T.   Mild congestive cardiac failure, no previous operations.

CASE U.   Similar pain 1 month ago. Had appendicectomy 1 year ago.

CASE V.   Cholecystectomy 1 year ago.

CASE W.   Rheumatic fever aged 15.

CASE X.   Indigestion for 3 months. Myocardial infarction 3 years ago.

CASE Y.   Nagging left iliac fossa pain and diarrhoea for 3 years.

CASE Z.   Nil relevant.

CASE A.   Mother had hiatus hernia.

CASE B.   Nil relevant.

CASE C.   Father and uncle have duodenal ulcers.

CASE D.   Nil relevant.

CASE E.   Mother had hysterectomy for fibroids.

CASE F.   Nil relevant.

CASE G.   Mother died of breast cancer.

CASE H.   Two members of the family ill with diarrhoea and vomiting at
present.

CASE I.   Nil relevant.

CASE J.   Brother had pyloric stenosis.

CASE K.   Sister had fibrocystic disease of the pancreas.

CASE L.   Mother has rheumatoid arthritis.

CASE M.   Father died of carcinoma of the rectum.

CASE N.   Two relatives have cystinuria.

CASE O.   One sister diabetic.

CASE P.   Brother has ankylosing spondylitis.

CASE Q.   Nil relevant.

CASE R.   Mother had gall-stones.

CASE S.   Nil relevant.

CASE T.   Mother had blood pressure.

CASE U.   Nil relevant.

CASE V.   Two relatives have had splenectomy.

CASE W.   Nil relevant.

CASE X.   Brother died of myocardial infarction.

CASE Y.   Nil relevant.

CASE Z.   Nil relevant.

	Temperature (°C)	Pulse (per minute)	Respiration (per minute)
CASE A.	39	100	20
CASE B.	36.5	120	30
CASE C.	37	100	30 – shallow
CASE D.	38.2	100	20
CASE E.	38	100	20
CASE F.	37.8	100	20
CASE G.	37	100	20
CASE H.	37.4	100	20
CASE I.	36.6	80	20
CASE J.	36.8	130	30
CASE K.	36	130	30
CASE L.	36.4	100	25
CASE M.	36.6	120	35

Other features on pages:

	Temperature (°C)	Pulse (per minute)	Respiration (per minute)
CASE N.	37	80	20
CASE O.	37	100	25
CASE P.	38	100	20
CASE Q.	39	100	20
CASE R.	37	100	20
CASE S.	36.2	140	35
CASE T.	36.8	100	25
CASE U.	37.6	80	20
CASE V.	37	90	20
CASE W.	37.8	110 A.F.	25
CASE X.	36	105	28
CASE Y.	38	110	30
CASE Z.	38	96	20

CASE A.   160/110

CASE B.   60/10

CASE C.   100/60

CASE D.   200/80

CASE E.   120/80

CASE F.   110/60

CASE G.   120/80

CASE H.   130/60

CASE I.   100/80

CASE J.   Not done.

CASE K.   Not done.

CASE L.   95/60

CASE M.   60/?

Other features on pages:

CASE N.	130/85
CASE O.	160/80
CASE P.	110/50
CASE Q.	120/80
CASE R.	130/80
CASE S.	Not done.
CASE T.	170/80
CASE U.	110/70
CASE V.	130/80
CASE W.	100/60
CASE X.	90/60
CASE Y.	100/70
CASE Z.	130/80

CASE A.	None.
CASE B.	None.
CASE C.	None.
CASE D.	Slight.
CASE E.	None.
CASE F.	None.
CASE G.	None.
CASE H.	Slight.
CASE I.	Sudden onset of gross massive distension.
CASE J.	None.
CASE K.	Marked distension.
CASE L.	None.
CASE M.	Slight.

CASE N.   None.

CASE O.   Marked distension.

CASE P.   Slight distension.

CASE Q.   None.

CASE R.   Moderate distension.

CASE S.   Slight distension.

CASE T.   Moderate distension.

CASE U.   None.

CASE V.   None.

CASE W.   None.

CASE X.   None.

CASE Y.   Slight distension.

CASE Z.   Slight lower abdominal distension.

CASE A.   Marked right upper quadrant tenderness.

CASE B.   Slight generalised tenderness. Tender particularly deep in the pelvis.

CASE C.   Tender all areas — especially epigastric and right iliac fossa.

CASE D.   Moderate tenderness in left iliac fossa.

CASE E.   Slightly tender suprapubically.

CASE F.   Tender in the right iliac fossa.

CASE G.   Mild epigastric tenderness.

CASE H.   Slight tenderness.

CASE I.   Slight generalised tenderness.

CASE J.   None.

CASE K.   None.

CASE L.   Very tender upper abdomen.

CASE M.   Very tender left ribs and generalised abdominal tenderness.

CASE N.   None.

CASE O.   None.

CASE P.   Slight generalised tenderness, maximum in the left iliac fossa.

CASE Q.   Slight right iliac fossa tenderness, radiating to the hypogastrium.

CASE R.   Slight generalised tenderness.

CASE S.   None.

CASE T.   Slight generalised tenderness, tender left groin.

CASE U.   Deep tenderness.

CASE V.   Slightly tender right upper quadrant.

CASE W.   Generalised tenderness, maximum in the left upper quadrant.

CASE X.   Widespread tenderness.

CASE Y.   Marked generalised tenderness.

CASE Z.   Very tender in the hypogastrium and left iliac fossa.

Other features on pages:

CASE A.   Marked guarding, no rigidity.

CASE B.   None.

CASE C.   Board-like rigidity.

CASE D.   Slight guarding.

CASE E.   Slight guarding.

CASE F.   Moderate guarding, no rigidity.

CASE G.   None.

CASE H.   None.

CASE I.   Slight guarding only.

CASE J.   None.

CASE K.   None.

CASE L.   Marked epigastric guarding, but not board-like rigidity.

CASE M.   Slight guarding left abdomen.

CASE N.   None.

CASE O.   Nonc.

CASE P.   None.

CASE Q.   Slight hypogastric and right iliac fossa guarding.

CASE R.   None.

CASE S.   None.

CASE T.   Slight guarding only.

CASE U.   Slight right iliac fossa guarding.

CASE V.   None.

CASE W.   Marked guarding left upper quadrant of abdomen with slight rigidity.

CASE X.   Widespread guarding with little rigidity.

CASE Y.   Marked generalised guarding, slight lower abdominal rigidity.

CASE Z.   Moderate guarding in left iliac fossa but no rigidity.

CASE A.   Possible mass palpable right upper quadrant.

CASE B.   None.

CASE C.   None.

CASE D.   Tender mass left iliac fossa.

CASE E.   None.

CASE F.   None.

CASE G.   None.

CASE H.   None.

CASE I.   None.

CASE J.   Sausage-shaped mass epigastrium.

CASE K.   None.

CASE L.   None.

CASE M.   None.

Other features on pages:

CASE N.   None.

CASE O.   Non-tender mass left iliac fossa.

CASE P.   None.

CASE Q.   None.

CASE R.   None.

CASE S.   None.

CASE T.   Tender mass left groin.

CASE U.   None.

CASE V.   Spleen palpable 3 fingers' breadth below costal margin.

CASE W.   None.

CASE X.   (?) Pulsatile upper abdominal mass.

CASE Y.   None.

CASE Z.   No mass palpable.

CASE A.   Normal.

CASE B.   Vaginal examination tender high on the right.

CASE C.   Normal.

CASE D.   Normal.

CASE E.   PV. Tender cervix and in both fornices.

CASE F.   Normal.

CASE G.   Clinically dehydrated, pelvic examination normal.

CASE H.   Normal.

CASE I.   Normal.

CASE J.   Normal.

CASE K.   Normal.

CASE L.   Patient shocked, vaginal examination small fibroids.

CASE M.   Shocked, mucosae very pale.

CASE N.   Normal.

CASE O.   Anaemic, vaginal examination normal.

CASE P.   Slightly anaemic.

CASE Q.   Acute follicular tonsillitis.

CASE R.   Vaginal examination normal, no hernias.

CASE S.   Mongol. Cardiac murmur, probably ASD.

CASE T.   Mild congestive failure.

CASE U.   Normal.

CASE V.   Slightly jaundiced.

CASE W.   Slight congestive failure, pan-systolic and early diastolic murmurs in
mitral area.

CASE X.   Left femoral pulse absent. Right femoral pulse has bruit.

CASE Y.   Shocked with blue periphery.

CASE Z.   Tender mass left fornix on vaginal examination.

CASE A.   Normal.

CASE B.   Present but few.

CASE C.   Absent.

CASE D.   Normal.

CASE E.   Normal.

CASE F.   Normal.

CASE G.   Increased and obstructive.

CASE H.   Hyperactive.

CASE I.   Hyperactive and tympanitic.

CASE J.   High pitched.

CASE K.   Hyperactive.

CASE L.   Present but few.

CASE M.   Absent.

Other features on pages:

CASE N.   Normal.

CASE O.   Obstructed and tinkling.

CASE P.   Hyperactive.

CASE Q.   Normal.

CASE R.   Borborygmi coincident with colic.

CASE S.   Hyperactive.

CASE T.   High pitched hyperactive bowel sounds.

CASE U.   Normal.

CASE V.   Normal.

CASE W.   Absent.

CASE X.   Absent.

CASE Y.   Absent.

CASE Z.   Normal.

CASE A.   Normal.

CASE B.   Tender high on the right.

CASE C.   Tender high anteriorly.

CASE D.   Normal.

CASE E.   Tender on both sides.

CASE F.   Tender on right.

CASE G.   Normal.

CASE H.   Slightly tender rectum, watery faeces, mucosa feels normal.

CASE I.   Normal.

CASE J.   No mass, little 'redcurrant jelly' on finger.

CASE K.   Normal.

CASE L.   Tender anteriorly.

CASE M.   Normal.

CASE N.　　　Normal.

CASE O.　　　Normal. Empty rectum.

CASE P.　　　Granular mucosa, loose blood-stained stool.

CASE Q.　　　Normal.

CASE R.　　　Normal.

CASE S.　　　Normal.

CASE T.　　　Normal.

CASE U.　　　Tender on the right.

CASE V.　　　Normal.

CASE W.　　　Slightly tender anteriorly.

CASE X.　　　Big prostate.

CASE Y.　　　Anterior tenderness.

CASE Z.　　　Tender anteriorly on the left side.

	Haemoglobin (g/100 ml)	WBCs (per mm^3)	ESR (mm in 1 hour)
CASE A.	14	21000 92% polymorphs	30
CASE B.	14	6000	5
CASE C.	15	4000	10
CASE D.	12	15000 80% polymorphs	35
CASE E.	12	16000	30
CASE F.	14	10000 76% polymorphs	20
CASE G.	16	5000	4
CASE H	14	9000	25
CASE I.	16	8000	10
CASE J.	12	6000	10
CASE K.	12	9000	20
CASE L.	16	6000	25
CASE M.	13.7	5000	5

	Haemoglobin (g/100 ml)	WBCs (per mm^3)	ESR (mm in 1 hour)
CASE N.	14	6200	20
CASE O.	7	6000	35
CASE P.	9	12000 72% polymorphs	38
CASE Q.	13.5	12500	25
CASE R.	13.6	5000	8
CASE S.	12	5000	5
CASE T.	16	3500	10
CASE U.	14	6000	10
CASE V.	13	5000	10

Blood film — spherocytosis. Reticulocyte count — 4%

	Haemoglobin (g/100 ml)	WBCs (per mm^3)	ESR (mm in 1 hour)
CASE W.	16	11000	30
CASE X.	13.4	11000	26
CASE Y.	16	12000	20
CASE Z.	14	11600	34

CASE A.   Solitary gall-stone visible on X-ray.

CASE B.   X-rays normal.

CASE C.   Air under the diaphragm on the right.

CASE D.   Normal.

CASE E.   Normal.

CASE F.   Normal.

CASE G.   Two dilated loops in the epigastrium showing valvulae conniventes.

CASE H.   Normal.

CASE I.   Grossly distended loop of the large bowel.

CASE J.   Some small-bowel distension with fluid levels.

CASE K.   Distended loop of small bowel containing some mottling.

CASE L.   'Sentinel loop'.

CASE M.   Normal.

CASE N.   Normal.

CASE O.   Marked dilatation of the bowel with fluid levels, caecum markedly
dilated.

CASE P.   Colon dilated round to the rectum.

CASE Q.   Normal.

CASE R.   Marked small-gut dilatation with fluid levels, (?) opacity in pelvis.

CASE S.   'Double bubble' sign.

CASE T.   Small-bowel distension with fluid levels.

CASE U.   Normal.

CASE V.   Normal.

CASE W.   Slight small bowel distension but no fluid levels.

CASE X.   Ring of calcification visible in expanded aorta.

CASE Y.   Generalised bowel dilatation. Erect films not done.

CASE Z.   (?) Opacity in the pelvis.

ACUTE ABDOMEN

CASE A.   Cholecystogram — gall-bladder not shown.

CASE B.   Peritoneal tap showed blood. Pregnancy test positive.

CASE C.   Amylase 80 somogyi units/100 ml.

CASE D.   Barium enema — marked spasm and diverticulosis.

CASE E.   High vaginal swab grew *Gonococcus.*

CASE F.   None done.

CASE G.   None done.

CASE H.   Stool culture grew *Shigella.*

CASE I.   None done.

CASE J.   Barium enema showed an ileocolic intussusception which was reduced spontaneously by the barium pressure.

CASE K.   None done.

CASE L.   Amylase 2000 somogyi units per 100 ml.

CASE M.   Peritoneal tap showed blood.

CASE N.   Urine — cystine crystals seen. IVP showed a filling defect in the lower left ureter.

CASE O.   Barium enema showed carcinoma of the sigmoid with almost complete obstruction.

CASE P.   Cultures negative. Barium enema showed gross total ulcerative colitis.

CASE Q.   None done.

CASE R.   None done.

CASE S.   None done.

CASE T.   None done.

CASE U.   None done.

CASE V.   Abnormal red cell frigidity curve. Subsequent intravenous cholangiogram showed dilated C.B.D.

CASE W.   None done.

CASE X.   None done.

CASE Y.   None done.

CASE Z.   None done.

CASE A.   *Acute cholecystitis*, settled on medical treatment. Cholecystectomy 6 weeks later.

CASE B.   *Ruptured ectopic pregnancy*. Laparotomy and removal of right tube (conservative surgery was not possible).

CASE C.   *Perforated duodenal ulcer*. Perforations sutured at laparotomy.

CASE D.   *Acute diverticulitis*. No operation necessary.

CASE E.   *Acute salpingitis*, resolved on antibiotics.

CASE F.   *Acute appendicitis*. Appendicectomy.

CASE G.   *Adhesion obstruction of the jejunum* from previous surgery. Division of adhesions at laparotomy.

CASE H.   *Acute gastro-enteritis*.

CASE I.   *Acute sigmoid volvulus*. Volvulus corrected after sigmoidoscopy and intubation. Patient later had a sigmoid colectomy.

CASE J.   *Intussusception* reduced spontaneously with barium enema.

CASE K.   *Meconium ileus*, required excision of loop of bowel most involved. Rest of small bowel washed out with enzymes.

CASE L.   *Acute pancreatitis*.

CASE M.   Laparotomy and splenectomy for *ruptured spleen*.

CASE N.   *Urinary calculus* passed spontaneously.

CASE O.   *Obstructing carcinoma of the colon*. Transverse colostomy and subsequent sigmoid colectomy.

CASE P.   *Severe ulcerative colitis*. Total proctocolectomy done as patient failed to respond to intensive medical treatment.

CASE Q.   *Mesenteric adenitis* in association with tonsillitis.

CASE R.   *Gall-stone ileus*. Gall-stone removed from obstructed terminal ileum. Subsequent cholecystectomy.

CASE S.   *Duodenal atresia* — gastroenterostomy.

CASE T.   *Strangulated left femoral hernia* — small segment of gangrenous ileum removed.

CASE U.   *Ruptured Graafian follicle*, free blood found in peritoneum.

CASE V.   *Pigment stones* in common bile duct due to *spherocytosis*. Stones removed from common bile duct, splenectomy performed.

CASE W.   *Splenic flexure infarction from embolus* in inferior mesenteric artery. Required resection of large bowel.

CASE X.   *Ruptured aortic aneurysm*. Dacron 'trouser graft' inserted.

CASE Y.   *Perforated diverticular disease* with faecal peritonitis. Diseased segment removed and proximal colostomy performed as too ill for anastomosis.

CASE Z.   *Infarcted twisted ovarian cyst*. As postmenopausal — hysterectomy and bilateral salpingo-oophorectomy performed.

ACUTE ABDOMEN

CASE A.   *Acute cholecystitis*. Notice the increasing constant pain in the right upper quadrant, also the radiation to the right scapula region. These patients frequently have nausea and vomiting. Notice the patient is obese and has had a history of indigestion for some years. Temperature is frequently higher than you find with appendicitis, and characteristically you find very marked, localised tenderness and guarding. In very early cases you may occasionally find a palpable gall-bladder. The white cells were raised, and unusually a gall-stone was seen on X-ray but this is only found in 10 per cent of cases. In this case the patient was treated medically and a cholecystectomy done six weeks later.

CASE B.   *Ruptured right tubal pregnancy*. Points to notice are the fact that she had nagging discomfort in the right iliac fossa for two days; this is due to colic in the expanding tube just prior to rupture. Then the pain became generalised. Notice too characteristically the radiation of the pain to the shoulder due to irritation of the diaphragm by blood. Note too the previous history of salpingitis. Notice the rapid pulse and low blood pressure. There was mild generalised tenderness but very little in the way of guarding. On pelvic examination notice the tenderness on the side of the ectopic. Notice too the reduced bowel sounds. The haemoglobin, in spite of frequently several litres of blood being in the peritoneal cavity, is of course still within normal limits as there has not been time for haemodilution. Peritoneal tap may be helpful, and a pregnancy test is usually positive.

CASE C.   *Perforated duodenal ulcer*. Features to notice are the age group and sex, the sudden onset of severe pain in the epigastrium. Notice the fact that the pain tends to become easier as the irritant fluid is diluted by peritoneal exudate. Note the radiation of pain to the shoulder and also to the right iliac fossa. This is due to fluid running down the paracolic gutter. Just occasionally most of the symptoms can be related to the right iliac fossa and mistaken for appendicitis. The past history of indigestion is helpful. Notice too the rapid shallow respiration due to irritation of the diaphragm and the board-like rigidity. The rectal tenderness is due to irritation of the peritoneum in the pouch of Douglas. Features that help separate this case from acute pancreatitis are the absence of back pain, the rigidity tends to be more board-like with a perforated ulcer, and repeated vomiting is more a feature of pancreatitis.

CASE D.   *Acute diverticulitis*. Notice the age group and long history of L.I.F. discomfort. There is no colic to suggest an obstructing lesion — which would indicate a carcinoma. The pyrexia suggests a true acute diverticulitis or pericolic abscess, and the diagnosis is supported by the tenderness and guarding in the left iliac fossa. Most carcinomas produce less tenderness but cannot be excluded on the clinical picture and the two conditions can of course coexist.

CASE E.   *Acute salpingitis*. The features that suggest this diagnosis are the lower abdominal pain and suprapubic tenderness, the history of a vaginal discharge, the temperature which is rather higher than found in appendicitis in this age group, and particularly the vaginal examination which shows tenderness on moving the cervix and in both fornices.

CASE F.   *Acute appendicitis*. This case shows the classical features of appendicitis. The central abdominal pain which tends to be colicky, moving to the right iliac fossa, the nausea, anorexia and constipation. Notice the slight frequency of micturition, which may imply irritation of the right ureter or bladder. A similar history of pain in the past is fairly common. Note the low fever, and the tenderness and guarding localised to the right iliac fossa. The rectal tenderness may suggest that the appendix lies fairly low, as in a pelvic appendicitis.

CASE G.   *Jejunal obstruction from adhesions* due to previous surgery. The features that suggest a very high small-bowel obstruction are the classical central colic, the onset of repeated vomiting very shortly after the pain started, the fact that the patient continues to pass flatus, the absence of distension, the rapid onset of clinical dehydration and the obstructive bowel sounds. There are only two common causes of small-bowel obstruction; these are adhesions from previous surgery or inflammation, and an obstructed hernia. The history of a previous gastrectomy for gastric ulcer makes the former likely, the other possibility being obstruction at the gastroduodenal anastomosis (the patient would probably have had a Billroth 1 gastrectomy if it was a gastric ulcer). The nature of the vomit may distinguish this, as in general obstruction the vomitus would contain bile. Abdominal X-ray helped to confirm that this was a jejunal obstruction, as the dilated loops of small bowel showed characteristic valvulae conniventes.

CASE H.   *Acute gastro-enteritis*. It is of course unusual for an acute gastro-enteritis to present as an acute abdomen, but just occasionally the features are suggestive of acute appendicitis and other conditions, particularly when there is marked colic, vomiting and tenderness. Appendicitis may also produce quite marked diarrhoea, particularly in children with an acute pelvic appendicitis. Features that suggest an acute gastro-enteritis are the marked diarrhoea, the family history or the history of contacts with similar diarrhoea, the absence of guarding or rigidity and the hyperactive bowel sound.

CASE I.   *Sigmoid volvulus*. This condition is unusual in this country although common in some parts of Africa. There is an increased incidence among in-patients of mental hospitals and most of these cases are elderly females. Features that strongly suggest closed-loop obstruction like a sigmoid volvulus is the sudden onset of gross massive distension. Occasionally one may get this story with carcinoma of the descending colon and a competent ileocaecal valve, when the whole of the colon will distend, but even so the distension is never as great as in these cases. The X-ray will show the characteristic features of a sigmoid volvulus. Notice that in this case it was possible to insert a lubricated rectal tube through a sigmoidoscope and deflate the sigmoid colon. If there are any signs of peritonitis, or if the patient's condition does not rapidly improve after this procedure, laparotomy is indicated.

CASE J.   *Intussusception*. Many intussusceptions occur between the age of 6 and 12 months. Notice that the child is completely well between bouts of colic. It is not unusual for a little blood or 'redcurrant jelly' to be passed *per rectum* or found on rectal examination. If a sausage-shaped mass is found, commonly in the upper abdomen, this clinches the diagnosis. Notice that the barium enema examination was successful in spontaneously reducing the intussusception. Many cases require laparotomy and operative reduction.

CASE K.   *Meconium ileus.* It is frequently difficult to separate the various causes in neonatal obstruction. Obviously in this case the family history of fibrocystic disease was useful. The fact that the child had passed a little meconium excluded anorectal atresia. A plain abdominal X-ray is frequently useful as there is a characteristic mottling due to inspissated meconium in many of these cases.

CASE L.   *Acute pancreatitis.* Features that help one make a diagnosis of acute pancreatitis are the sudden onset of severe upper abdominal pain radiating into the back, the repeated vomiting, a prior history suggestive of gall-stone disease, marked epigastric guarding without board-like rigidity. The fact that the patient was female makes the diagnosis of a perforated peptic ulcer less likely. Notice the so-called 'sentinel loop' on plain abdominal X-ray. This is due to local ileus around the inflamed pancreas. The amylase of 2000 somogyi units clinches the diagnosis.

CASE M.   *Ruptured spleen.* Ruptured spleen is the commonest cause of marked intraperitoneal bleeding after an accident. The features that suggest the diagnosis are unexplained shock after a road traffic accident, and the likelihood of ruptured spleen is supported by the tenderness of the left ribs and left upper abdomen. Notice the radiation of the pain to the left shoulder and the positive peritoneal tap.

CASE N.   *Left ureteric colic.* Most cases of ureteric colic show the classical features of pain radiating from the loin down to the groin, but notice the atypical features of this case in that most of the pain was in the left flank and left iliac fossa. Repeated vomiting is fairly common, and, if asked, most patients will admit to slight frequency and dysuria. Most cases with ureteric stone show a calculus on plain abdominal X-ray. This case was rare in that the cause of the ureteric colic was cystinuria. The stones are not seen on a plain film.

CASE O.   *Obstructing carcinoma of the sigmoid colon.* Features to note are the age group, the previous bowel history and weight loss, the symptoms suggestive of large-bowel obstruction, that is hypogastric colic, marked distension, pain going on for two days but without vomiting, and 3-day history of constipation. The fact that the patient is still passing flatus suggests that it is an incomplete obstruction. The finding of a non-tender mass in the left iliac fossa, although unusual, clinches the diagnosis.

CASE P.   *Acute ulcerative colitis.* It is rare for ulcerative colitis to present as an acute abdomen, but about 5 per cent of cases present in this way as an acute fulminating colitis. Features that suggest the diagnosis are the passage of blood and mucus with the diarrhoea, and the rectal findings of a granular mucosa with loose blood-stained stools.

278

CASE Q.　　*Acute mesenteric adenitis*. This condition is commonly mistaken for acute appendicitis, although in this case the diagnosis is made somewhat easier by the fact that the girl had had an appendicectomy two years previously! The features that distinguish mesenteric adenitis from appendicitis are the following. (1) The pain tends to start in the right iliac fossa and does not have the characteristic shift from the central abdomen. (2) The history of a sore throat. Many cases of mesenteric adenitis have enlarged cervical glands. This girl had an associated acute follicular tonsillitis. (3) The temperature tends to be higher with mesenteric adenitis. (4) Sometimes one can detect that the site of maximum tenderness moves with different postures.

CASE R.　　*Gall-stone ileus*. Notice that the pain preceded the onset of repeated vomiting by 4 hours. Notice the central colic and moderate abdominal distension. Notice too that the pain has been going on for 10 hours but the vomiting for only 6 hours, but that the vomiting has been repeated. The relation of the onset of vomiting to the onset of pain gives some indication of the level of the obstruction. The previous history of acute cholecystitis and the absence of the two common causes of small-bowel obstruction (that is hernia or previous surgery), should make one suspicious. It is not rare to be able to see the gall-stone on a plain abdominal film, usually in the pelvis as it tends to stick at the terminal ileum.

CASE S.　　*Duodenal atresia*. This is obviously one of the neonatal intestinal obstructions again. The features that may suggest a duodenal stenosis or atresia are that the baby failed to pass meconium, the fact that there is a higher incidence of duodenal atresia in Mongols and the finding of the characteristic 'double bubble' sign on plain abdominal X-ray.

CASE T.　　*Strangulated left femoral hernia*. Most cases of strangulated hernia are obvious, as most of the pain is localised to the hernia, and the abdominal symptoms and signs develop later. However, one may be caught out, particularly in the elderly and obese. Note the features of small bowel obstruction — central abdominal colic, repeated vomiting, abdominal distension and absolute constipation. In these cases one should always search carefully at the femoral rings.

CASE U.　　*Ruptured Graafian follicle*. This case is frequently mistaken for appendicitis. The features that suggest a midcycle bleed (Mittelschmerz) are the onset of pain in one iliac fossa, the absence of anorexia, the history of previous bouts of similar pain, and the relationship to the menstrual cycle. Guarding is usually absent or mild, and the white cells not raised.

CASE V.　　*Common duct pigment stones secondary to spherocytosis*. This is a rare case but of clinical interest. Notice the right upper quadrant severe pain and radiation to the scapula. Common duct pathology rarely produces colic but frequently is associated with jaundice. The features that suggest an underlying cause for the gall-stones such as an haemolytic anaemia are the family history of splenectomy and the palpable spleen. The findings are confirmed by blood film and abnormal red cell fragility. This patient's exploration of common bile duct was combined with splenectomy.

CASE W.   *Mesenteric embolism*. Although this case is rare, one should always be suspicious of patients with an acute abdomen who also show atrial fibrillation. Most cases of mesenteric embolism affect the small bowel. In this case the splenic flexure of the large bowel was involved, and the embolus was in the inferior mesenteric artery. The features that suggest a vascular crisis as a cause for the acute abdomen are the sudden onset of continuous pain, the passage of some dark blood and the marked guarding which may be out of proportion to the other clinical signs. The white-cell count may be very high, though it was not in this case. The absence of bowel sounds suggests a serious crisis inside the abdomen.

CASE X.   *Ruptured aortic aneurysm*. Note that the patient is an elderly male. Notice the sudden onset of central abdominal pain becoming generalised and also radiating to the back. One should not be fooled by the history of indigestion into thinking that this is a perforated ulcer. There is a higher incidence of peptic ulcers in patients with aneurysms. The previous history of a myocardial infarction suggests he has generalised arteriosclerosis. On careful examination in most cases one is able to detect a pulsatile abdominal mass, although the severity of the guarding and rigidity may preclude this. Sometimes absence of the femoral pulses is present. In the majority of cases plain abdominal film will demonstrate calcification in the wall of the aneurysm.

CASE Y.   *Faecal peritonitis from perforated diverticulum*. Features to note in this case are that the pain started suddenly in the left iliac fossa and became generalised. There is a previous history suggestive of diverticular disease, that is nagging discomfort in the left iliac fossa and episodes of diarrhoea for the previous three years. Patients with faecal peritonitis frequently become very ill quickly, and the clinical features of shock and cyanosis may suggest this. Most of the rigidity was in the lower abdomen and this may suggest the diagnosis. One may mistake this condition for a perforated peptic ulcer or a perforated appendix, which frequently produce atypical features in the elderly.

CASE Z.   *Twisted ovarian cyst*. Features that suggest this case are the sudden onset of pain in the iliac fossa. If it is on the left side in a patient who is rather young for a complication of diverticular disease, it makes the diagnosis somewhat easier. Notice the very gross local tenderness and guarding without any generalised abdominal signs. One is dependent upon detecting the mass on bimanual examination.

SECTION 5

Cryptic cases A to Z

Try your skill at deciphering these interesting and unusual surgical cases. Select the clinical features that you think are important, and score according to the number of pages you turn to arrive at a correct diagnosis. Deduct your total from 25 for final score.

Case	U.G.	P.G.	Case	U.G.	P.G.
A	8	11	N	11	14
B	9	12	O	10	13
C	10	13	P	11	14
D	10	13	Q	12	15
E	10	13	R	12	15
F	11	14	S	13	16
G	9	12	T	10	13
H	8	11	U	9	12
I	7	10	V	10	13
J	10	13	W	13	16
K	11	14	X	9	12
L	12	15	Y	10	13
M	12	15	Z	13	16

CASE A.   Man, aged 36, complaining of a lump in the neck.

CASE B.   Female, aged 56, complaining of shortness of breath.

CASE C.   Female, aged 65, complaining of bleeding *per rectum* for 8 hours.

CASE D.   Female, aged 54, complaining of pain in the right shoulder for 1 week.

CASE E.   Male, aged 64, complaining of pain in the legs for 3 days.

CASE F.   Female, aged 56, complaining of shortness of breath and food sticking for 1 month.

CASE G.   Male, aged 42, complaining of fever and a swelling in the left scrotum.

CASE H.   Male, aged 19, complaining of abdominal pain for 19 hours.

CASE I.   Girl, aged 19, complaining of right iliac fossa pain for 30 hours.

CASE J.   Male, aged 34, complaining of pain in the back for 2 weeks.

CASE K.   Female, aged 52, complaining of lump in both groins and tiredness.

CASE L.   Female, aged 43, complaining of diarrhoea for 3 months.

CASE M.   Male, aged 72, vomiting for 1 week.

Other features will be found on pages:

CASE N.   Male, aged 58, complaining of increasing deafness in the left ear.

CASE O.   Male, aged 41, complaining of cough and ache in the right loin.

CASE P.   Male, aged 34, complaining of cough, backache and weakness of the
legs.

CASE Q.   Female, aged 47, with sudden onset paralysis left side.

CASE R.   Male, aged 62, with fits.

CASE S.   Male, aged 27, with cough and dysphagia for 6 weeks.

CASE T.   Male, aged 7, with central abdominal colic and vomiting for 6 hours.

CASE U.   34 year-old female in coma for 6 hours.

CASE V.   Male, aged 67, with right lower chest pain for 6 weeks.

CASE W.   Male, aged 3, with malaise and abdominal distension.

CASE X.   Female, aged 54, with swelling of the right parotid, cough, and a
rash on the legs.

CASE Y.   Male, aged 71, with back pain for 3 months.

CASE Z.   Male, aged 61, with haematemesis.

CASE A.   Lump in the left supraclavicular fossa region for 6 weeks. Painless, gradually increasing in size.

CASE B.   Increasing shortness of breath on exercise, palpitations and ankle oedema for 4 months.

CASE C.   Profuse bright red bleeding *per rectum* for 8 hours. Blood loss, (?) 2 pints, now complains of weakness.

CASE D.   Sudden onset of pain in the right shoulder 1 week ago, continuous nagging pain increased by moving the arm.

CASE E.   Sudden onset pain in the right calf 3 days ago, 2 days ago developed pain in the left thigh.

CASE F.   Increasing dysphagia for 1 month, can now only swallow fluids. Food sticks at the level of the lower neck.

CASE G.   Recurrent attacks of fever and sweating for 4 weeks. Painless swelling of the left scrotum for 1 week.

CASE H.   Nineteen hours ago developed generalised colic, pain moved to the left iliac fossa 6 hours ago and is now constant.

CASE I.   Continuous nagging right iliac fossa pain for 30 hours with occasional colic.

CASE J.   Increasing aching discomfort in the right loin for 2 weeks.

CASE K.   Swelling in the left groin for 6 months, which appears on standing and goes down at night-time. Painless continuous swelling in the right groin for 4 weeks.

CASE L.   Increasing bouts of diarrhoea for 3 months, usually sudden onset, watery brown diarrhoea with no blood or mucus. Attacks last 1 or 2 days.

CASE M.   Generally ill for 2 months with anorexia, nausea and weight loss. Bouts of vomiting for the last week with hiccups and foul taste in the mouth.

CASE N.   Gradually increasing deafness in the left ear for 8 months, now completely deaf in that ear.

CASE O.   Increasing ache in the right loin for 1 month, intermittent tickling cough for 1 month.

CASE P.   Ill for one year with malaise, fever and cough. Increasing lower thoracic backache 1 month, weakness and paraesthesia in both legs for 1 week.

CASE Q.   History from husband, patient was washing up today when suddenly complained of headache and then blacked out and collapsed on the floor.

CASE R.   About 5 grand mal epileptic fits in the last 24 hours, each lasting about 5 minutes. Complains of some headache in between.

CASE S.   Gradually increasing dysphagia for 6 weeks, worse with solid food which appears to stick in the midsternal region, tickling cough worse at night, no sputum.

CASE T.   Well until 6 hours ago, when gradual onset of central abdominal colic and has vomited 3 times.

CASE U.   Sudden onset of severe pain in the occipital region, then rapidly became unconscious.

CASE V.   Increasing dull constant ache in the right lower chest radiating to the right upper quadrant of the abdomen for the last 6 weeks.

CASE W.   Child unwell for 3 months, general malaise, anorexia and weight loss. Abdomen enlarging.

CASE X.   Painless swelling in the right parotid region for 1 month. Recent unproductive cough, worse at night. Rash on the legs for 2 days.

CASE Y.   Increasing constant backache in the upper lumbar region for 3 months, worse on moving or coughing.

CASE Z.   Well until 6 hours ago, when vomited 1½ litres of bright red blood.

CASE A.   Barman, smokes 30 cigarettes a day. Two members of his family have ileostomies.

CASE B.   Mother had a goitre, housewife.

CASE C.   Housewife, mother has gall-stones.

CASE D.   Mother and sister died of breast cancer.

CASE E.   Clerk. No relevant family history. Smokes 20 cigarettes a day.

CASE F.   Mother had renal stones.

CASE G.   Irish labourer. Smokes 50 cigarettes a day. Drinks heavily. Father died carcinoma of the bronchus.

CASE H.   Builder. Smokes 20 cigarettes a day. Father died of myocardial infarction. Mother has diverticular disease.

CASE I.   Mother had breast cancer.

CASE J.   Father had duodenal ulcer. Carpenter, smokes 35 cigarettes a day.

CASE K.   Nil relevant.

CASE L.   Mother had breast cancer.

CASE M.   Mother diabetic. Retired carpenter, smokes 30 cigarettes a day.

CASE N.   Brother and uncle have nerve tumours.

CASE O.   Father had tuberculosis. Electrical fitter, smokes 20 cigarettes a day.

CASE P.   Nil relevant.

CASE Q.   Two aunts had kidney trouble and died in middle age. Housewife, smokes 15 cigarettes a day.

CASE R.   Steelworker, smokes 40 cigarettes a day for most of his life. No relevant family history.

CASE S.   Non-smoker. Works as a car mechanic. No family history.

CASE T.   Nil relevant.

CASE U.   Mother has heart failure. Father died of myocardial infarction. Housewife, smokes 30 cigarettes a day.

CASE V.   No relevant family history. Retired Australian sheep farmer. Has been in England for 3 years. Non-smoker.

CASE W.   Mother diabetic.

CASE X.   Mother had gastric ulcer. Father died of bronchitis. Housewife with 3 children. Non-smoker.

CASE Y.   Father died carcinoma of the bronchus, mother died of carcinoma of the breast. Retired postman, smokes 20 cigarettes a day.

CASE Z.   Nil relevant in family history. Steel erector, heavy drinker and smokes 30 cigarettes a day.

CASE A.   'Piles' for many years. Nil else.

CASE B.   Goitre for 20 years.

CASE C.   Left iliac-fossa discomfort on and off for 3 years. Had a deep vein thrombosis 6 weeks ago. Is on Warfarin.

CASE D.   Partial gastrectomy for duodenal ulceration 7 years ago.

CASE E.   Myocardial infarction 4 years ago.

CASE F.   Menorrhagia for 3 years.

CASE G.   Pulmonary tuberculosis aged 12. Had chemotherapy for 2 years.

CASE H.   Similar pain 2 years ago, which subsided in 24 hours.

CASE I.   Tonsillectomy aged 6.

CASE J.   Continuous ache in the left tibial region for 2 months. Appendicectomy aged 10.

CASE K.   No past medical history.

CASE L.   Appendicectomy, hysterectomy aged 38 for fibroids.

CASE M.   Polya gastrectomy for duodenal ulcer 10 years ago. Right inguinal herniography.

CASE N.   Nil relevant.

CASE O.   Fracture left tibia 2 years ago.

CASE P.   Nil relevant.

CASE Q.   Occasional headaches and dizziness in the past, recurrent cystitis.

CASE R.   Kidney stones aged 50. Had an operation on the left kidney.

CASE S.   Appendicectomy aged 7.

CASE T.   Allergic to milk and eggs.

CASE U.   On phenobarbitone and epanutin for epilepsy 5 years.

CASE V.   Pneumonia aged 52. Left inguinal hernia repair aged 60.

CASE W.   Recurrent tonsillitis.

CASE X.   Hysterectomy for fibroids aged 42.

CASE Y.   Cholecystectomy aged 50.

CASE Z.   Some indigestion for 6 months, on Indomethacin for pain in the right hip on walking 4 months.

CRYPTIC CASES

CASE A.　　　Weight loss 2 stones in 1 year. Has been passing blood and mucus *per rectum* for 6 months. Is now short of breath on climbing stairs. No diarrhoea.

CASE B.　　　Weight loss 2 stones, spontaneous attacks of palpitations, admits to being anxious and jumpy, no cough.

CASE C.　　　Occasional diarrhoea, no previous bleeding *per rectum*, bruises easily.

CASE D.　　　Short of breath on climbing stairs, weight loss 8 lbs in last 3 months, nauseated, gets headaches.

CASE E.　　　Pain deep in the right calf but near the surface on the left thigh. Describes it as a burning pain. Has had some indigestion for last 6 months, and has lost 1 stone in weight.

CASE F.　　　Short of breath on climbing 6 stairs, has lost 1 stone in weight, complains of soreness in the mouth.

CASE G.　　　Cough with white sputum, some vague left abdominal pain unrelated to meals, one episode of haematuria.

CASE H.　　　Anorexic, has vomited once, constipated.

CASE I.　　　Nausea, no vomiting, not anorexic, bowels regular, some frequency and dysuria.

CASE J.　　　Gradually increasing loin ache, constant night and day, with occasional radiation to right groin. Indigestion for 6 weeks — epigastric discomfort after meals.

CASE K.　　　Increasing tiredness and lethargy for 4 weeks, right groin swelling has gradually enlarged, the left groin lump increases in size on coughing. Menopause 3 years ago.

CASE L.　　　Little short of breath on exercise, says she flushes easily particularly after alcohol. Some abdominal colic, and has lost weight over the last 3 months. Little ankle oedema.

CASE M.　　　Vomit bile-stained but not projectile, no haematemesis. Nocturia for the last year, increasing, now 4 times a night. Some dribbling incontinence for last month. No haematuria. No cough, abdominal pain or distension. Weight loss

1 stone in last 2 months. Some bleeding *per rectum* for 2 weeks, associated with diarrhoea.

CASE N.   No problems with balance, did have tinnitus at onset of deafness, some headache on the left side of the head, no diplopia.

CASE O.   Constant dull ache in the right loin which is getting worse. Unproductive cough, especially at night-time. Weight loss half a stone in 2 months.

CASE P.   Cough, worse at night, with greenish sputum. Occasional haemoptysis. Constant lower thoracic back pain, worse on coughing and movement. Legs weak. Weight loss 1 stone.

CASE Q.   Occasional occipital headaches when under stress, no previous blackouts, no paraesthesia.

CASE R.   Some personality change over the last 3 months. Frequent headaches, vomited twice yesterday. Frequent cough and sputum, especially in the mornings.

CASE S.   Weight loss 3 lbs over 6 weeks, some itching and sweating.

CASE T.   Anorexic for 6 hours, bowels regular, no diarrhoea or bleeding.

CASE U.   Direct questioning impossible.

CASE V.   Some anorexia and nausea, weight loss 6 lbs over the last 6 weeks, no vomiting, no bleeding *per rectum*, no cough or dyspnoea.

CASE W.   No vomiting, no pain, no bleeding *per rectum*, 1 episode of haematuria 1 month ago.

CASE X.   Swelling in the left parotid region, does not alter with food, no sputum or haemoptysis, well otherwise.

CASE Y.   No weakness or paraesthesia of the legs, no cough, appetite poor and has lost 1 stone in weight. No vomiting, bowels regular with no bleeding *per rectum*.

CASE Z.   No previous nausea or vomiting, no melaena or bleeding *per rectum*, no abdominal pain apart from indigestion which is epigastric and only occurs half an hour after meals, and is promptly relieved by antacids. Bowels open regularly, micturition normal.

CASE A.   Anaemic, apyrexial, cachetic, thyroid normal, hard node left axilla.

CASE B.   Thin, nervous lady, not anaemic, breasts normal, no lymphadeno-pathy.

CASE C.   Not anaemic, shocked and sweating, thirsty, multiple bruises on the arms.

CASE D.   Lymph nodes left axilla, hard lump 4 cm x 2 cm in left breast adherent to the skin and breast wall.

CASE E.   Slightly anaemic, lymph node left supraclavicular fossa (firm, 1 cm diameter), (?) slightly jaundiced.

CASE F.   Markedly anaemic, angular stomatitis, koilonychia.

CASE G.   Fit, not anaemic, temperature 38 °C, no lymphadenopathy.

CASE H.   Temperature 37.8 °C, flushed, not anaemic, no glands.

CASE I.   Fit girl, not anaemic, no glands, temperature 39.8 °C.

CASE J.   Looks fit, not anaemic, no lymphadenopathy, breasts normal.

CASE K.   Slightly anaemic, enlarged nodes right axilla, apyrexial.

CASE L.   Looks flushed but apyrexial and not anaemic.

CASE M.   Pale, lethargic, sallow complexion.

CASE N.   Fit, 58-year old, not anaemic, slight kyphoscoliosis, some brown patches on back 1 cm in diameter — coffee coloured.

CASE O.   Looks fit, no glands.

CASE P.   Thin, ill man, apyrexial, slight kyphoscoliosis and tenderness over the spines of T9–11.

CASE Q.   Unconscious but responds to painful stimuli, total left hemiplegia, not anaemic.

CASE R.   Looks fit, slightly drowsy. Not clinically anaemic.

CASE S.   (?) Slightly anaemic, several enlarged nodes right supraclavicular fossa, slightly rubbery consistency. Temperature 38 °C.

CASE T.   Fit, flushed child, temperature 37.4 °C.

CASE U.   Arched back and neck, stertorus breathing, not clinically anaemic.

CASE V.   Thin, slightly wasted, temperature 38 °C, not clinically anaemic, (?) tinge of jaundice.

CASE W.   Sick, thin child, apyrexial.

CASE X.   Looks fit, not anaemic.

CASE Y.   Anaemic, thin, obviously in pain.

CASE Z.   Pale, sweating, apyrexial.

CASE A.   Mass left supraclavicular fossa, firm and fixed 3 cm x 2 cm in diameter, not attached to the skin.

CASE B.   Mild exophthalmos, multinodular goitre.

CASE C.   Subconjunctival haemorrhage right eye.

CASE D.   Normal.

CASE E.   Some foetor oris.

CASE F.   Firm gland right lower jugular chain.

CASE G.   Few spider naevi.

CASE H.   Port-wine naevus left face.

CASE I.   Pre-auricular sinus.

CASE J.   Normal, no goitre.

CASE K.   Firm node right anterior triangle, no goitre.

CASE L.   Normal.

CASE M.   Foul 'uriniferous' breath, very dry, thyroid normal, no glands.

CASE N.   Mouth normal, neck normal, right ear normal, nerve deafness almost complete left ear, slight left facial weakness, no papilloedema.

CASE O.   Normal.

CASE P.   Few shotty nodes in the neck, mucosae slightly pale.

CASE Q.   Head and eyes deviated to the right.

CASE R.   Left supraclavicular node.

CASE S.   Several enlarged nodes in the right supraclavicular fossa, slightly rubbery but still mobile and not attached to the skin.

CASE T.   Normal.

CASE U.   Port-wine naevus right face and mouth. Neck stiffness ++.

CASE V.   Normal.

CASE W.   Normal.

CASE X.   Diffuse soft enlargement of both parotids, the right greater than the left. Few cervical nodes in the right neck.

CASE Y.   Normal.

CASE Z.   Few spider naevi on the face.

CASE A.   Pulse 100, sinus rhythm, BP 110/60, apex beat displaced to the left, heart sounds — systolic ejection murmur.

CASE B.   Pulse 160, atrial fibrillation, BP 110/70, JVP raised 2 cm, apex beat not displaced, no murmurs, moderate ankle oedema.

CASE C.   Pulse 110 regular, BP 80/40, JVP not raised, heart sounds normal.

CASE D.   Pulse 72 regular, BP 130/80, heart sounds normal, apex beat displaced to the left.

CASE E.   Pulse 82 regular, BP 200/110, apex beat displaced thrusting, JVP not raised, no murmurs.

CASE F.   Pulse 100, BP 110/80, JVP raised 2 cm, apex beat not displaced, no murmurs.

CASE G.   Pulse 100 regular, BP 130/80, no murmurs.

CASE H.   Pulse 100, BP 120/80, no murmurs.

CASE I.   Pulse 100 regular, BP 120/80, heart sounds normal.

CASE J.   Pulse 80 regular, BP 130/80, heart sounds normal.

CASE K.   Pulse 64 regular, BP 140/80, heart sounds normal.

CASE L.   Pulse 60 regular, BP 135/80, apex beat right ventricular heave, systolic murmur maximum in the tricuspid area.

CASE M.   Pulse 110 regular, BP 180/115, apex beat displaced to the left, heart sounds — faint pericardial friction rub, no murmurs.

CASE N.   Pulse 80 regular, BP 160/90, apex beat normal, heart sounds normal.

CASE O.   Pulse 80 regular, BP 120/80, heart sounds normal.

CASE P.   Pulse 86 regular, BP 120/70, heart sounds normal.

CASE Q.   Pulse 92 regular, BP 190/120, apex beat displaced to anterior
axillary line. Left ventricular hypertrophy. No murmurs.

CASE R.   Pulse 72 regular, BP 130/80, heart sounds normal.

CASE S.   Pulse 70 regular, BP 110/70, heart sounds normal.

CASE T.   Pulse 106 regular, BP 110/70, heart sounds normal.

CASE U.   Pulse 100 regular, BP 190/110, heart sounds normal.

CASE V.   Pulse 100, BP 160/80, apex beat not displaced, heart sounds normal.

CASE W.   Pulse 92 regular, BP 170/95, apex beat normal, heart sounds normal,
no murmurs.

CASE X.   Pulse 80 regular, BP 135/80, heart sounds normal.

CASE Y.   Pulse 100 regular, BP 160/90, apex beat displaced to the left, early
systolic murmur at the apex.

CASE Z.   Pulse 120 regular, BP 90/60, heart sounds normal.

CASE A.   Trachea central, reduced air entry in the bases, bilateral basal creps.

CASE B.   Normal.

CASE C.   Normal.

CASE D.   Trachea shifted to the left, reduced air entry right base, percussion note stony dull right base, no air entry right base.

CASE E.   Slightly hyper-resonant, few scattered rhonchi.

CASE F.   Normal.

CASE G.   Trachea deviated to the right, percussion note increased right apex, bronchial breathing and reduced air entry with increased vocal fremitus right apex. No added sounds.

CASE H.   Trachea central, percussion note slightly reduced left base, absent liver dullness on the right.

CASE I.   Normal.

CASE J.   Chest clear.

CASE K.   Normal.

CASE L.   Few creps in both bases.

CASE M.   Trachea central, reduced air entry and percussion note in the bases with bilateral basal crepitations.

CASE N.   Normal.

CASE O.   Normal, apart from occasional creps which appear on coughing.

CASE P.   Trachea central, air entry full, normal percussion note, few coarse creps in the right apex.

CASE Q.   Lung fields clear.

CASE R.   Normal.

CASE S.   Normal.

CASE T.   Chest clear.

CASE U.   Normal.

CASE V.   Trachea central, reduced percussion note right base, reduced air entry right base, breath sounds vesicular, no added sounds.

CASE W.   Chest clear.

CASE X.   Lung fields clear.

CASE Y.   Few creps in bases, otherwise normal.

CASE Z.   Hyper-resonant chest and expiratory wheeze.

CASE A.   Firm mobile mass in the left iliac fossa 4 cm x 5 cm, liver enlarged 2 finger breadths and is irregular.

CASE B.   Liver enlarged 1 finger breadth, smooth, slightly tender, no spleno-megaly or other masses.

CASE C.   Tender left iliac fossa, (?) vague mass.

CASE D.   Liver enlarged 3 finger breadths, irregular, firm and non-tender.

CASE E.   Slightly tender in the epigastric region, (?) mass.

CASE F.   Normal.

CASE G.   Mass left upper quadrant, palpable bimanually, liver enlarged 2 finger breadths, smooth, varicocoele left scrotum.

CASE H.   Tender in the left iliac fossa with guarding and rebound tenderness.

CASE I.   Slightly tender mass in the right iliac fossa, no guarding, bowel sounds normal.

CASE J.   Mass in the right upper quadrant, palpable bimanually, moves on respiration, slightly tender.

CASE K.   Irregular hepatomegaly 3 finger breadths, no ascites, no spleen or kidney palpable, reducible left inguinal hernia, 3 firm nodes 2 cm in diameter in the right groin. These nodes are fixed.

CASE L.   Liver enlarged 2 finger breadths, firm edge, abdomen distended, increased bowel sounds, no abdominal masses apart from liver.

CASE M.   Liver and kidneys not palpable, scars from duodenal ulcer operation and hernia operation, bladder palpable above the umbilicus.

CASE N.   Normal.

CASE O.   Palpable right kidney which is slightly enlarged, possible pelvic mass, absent right testis ('since birth').

CASE P.   Normal.

CASE Q.   Bilateral irregular masses in the upper abdomen palpable bimanually, slight hepatomegaly.

CASE R.   Slight hepatomegaly.

CASE S.   Spleen enlarged 3 finger breadths, liver normal, no other masses.

CASE T.   Vague generalised tenderness, no guarding or rigidity, bowel sounds normal.

CASE U.   Normal.

CASE V.   Liver enlarged 3 finger breadths slightly tender and irregular.

CASE W.   Markedly distended by smooth solid mass occupying most of the abdomen and dull to percussion.

CASE X.   Normal.

CASE Y.   Normal.

CASE Z.   Liver enlarged 2 finger breadths, spleen just palpable and is firm, no ascites.

CASE A.   Multiple rectal polyps palpable, mucus +, blood +, mucosa not granular.

CASE B.   Small haemorrhoids, otherwise normal.

CASE C.   Fresh blood, no masses; vaginal examination — small fibroids.

CASE D.   Firm anterior shelf in the pouch of Douglas.

CASE E.   Normal.

CASE F.   Normal.

CASE G.   Normal.

CASE H.   Tender on rectal examination high on the left.

CASE I.   Normal.

CASE J.   Normal.

CASE K.   Normal. Uterus not enlarged.

CASE L.   Normal.

CASE M.   Moderately enlarged benign prostate, rectal mucosa normal.

CASE N.   Normal.

CASE O.   Normal.

CASE P.   Normal.

CASE Q.   Normal.

CASE R.   Prostate slightly enlarged.

CASE S.   Normal.

CASE T.   Normal.

CASE U.   Normal.

CASE V.   Slightly enlarged prostate.

CASE W.   Lower border of mass just palpable.

CASE X.   Normal.

CASE Y.   Prostate slightly enlarged, but soft.

CASE Z.   Normal.

CASE A.   Slight pitting oedema of ankles.

CASE B.   Hands warm and sweaty, moderate ankle oedema.

CASE C.   Multiple bruises, right calf swollen and tender.

CASE D.   Right shoulder swollen, not hot, some crepitus and a lot of pain on movement. All movements grossly limited.

CASE E.   Right calf hot, swollen and tender. Left thigh tender red line along superficial long saphenous vein.

CASE F.   Koilonychia.

CASE G.   Lateral palms slightly red, slight tremor.

CASE H.   Normal.

CASE I.   Normal.

CASE J.   Slight swelling left tibia, near the knee, not tender and no increased temperature over the bone. Full movements of all joints.

CASE K.   Darkly pigmented raised lesion 1.5 cm in diameter on the sole of the right foot.

CASE L.   Slight ankle oedema.

CASE M.   Slight ankle oedema.

CASE N.   Few spindle-shaped subcutaneous nodules on both arms. These are slightly tender, and pressure produces some paraesthesia down the arms.

CASE O.   Normal.

CASE P.   Normal.

CASE Q.   Slight ankle oedema.

CASE R.   Clubbing of the fingers.

CASE S.   Scratch marks on the legs.

CASE T.   Purpuric rash on the legs with some red blotches and a few urticarial lesions.

CASE U.   Normal.

CASE V.   Normal.

CASE W.   Slight ankle oedema.

CASE X.   Erythema nodosum on the legs.

CASE Y.   Right ankle oedema.

CASE Z.   Liver palms and slight flapping tremor.

CASE A.   Normal.

CASE B.   Normal.

CASE C.   Normal.

CASE D.   Normal.

CASE E.   Normal.

CASE F.   Normal.

CASE G.   Normal.

CASE H.   Normal.

CASE I.   Normal.

CASE J.   Normal.

CASE K.   Normal.

CASE L.   Normal.

CASE M.   Lethargic and drowsy, no focal neurological signs.

Other features will be found on pages:

CASE N.   Slight left facial weakness, no papilloedema, slight reduction left corneal reflex.

CASE O.   Normal.

CASE P.   Generalised weakness of both legs, reduced sensation to touch and pinprick below T11.

CASE Q.   Left plantar response extensor, total left hemiplegia.

CASE R.   Papilloedema, no focal neurological lesion apart from some weakness of the left 6th nerve.

CASE S.   Normal.

CASE T.   Normal.

CASE U.   In coma. Only just responds to painful stimuli. No focal neurological signs.

CASE V.   Normal.

CASE W.   Normal.

CASE X.   Normal.

CASE Y.   Tender upper lumbar spine, some limitation of all movements by pain, no focal neurological signs.

CASE Z.   Slightly confused and disorientated, no focal neurological signs.

Other features will be found on pages:

CASE A.   Haemoglobin (Hb) 5 g (per 100 ml), PCV 28, MCV 68, MCHC 29, WBCs 5600, ESR 35.

CASE B.   Hb 13.6 g, WBCs 7600, ESR 25, film and platelets normal.

CASE C.   Hb 13 g, film normal, WBCs 7900, ESR 4, platelets 264 000.

CASE D.   Hb 11.5 g, MCHC 32, PCV 42, WBCs 3200, ESR 25.

CASE E.   Hb 10.6, MCHC 29.6, PCV 39, WBCs 3600, ESR 84.

CASE F.   Hb 5 g, MCHC 24, PCV 30, MCV 66, WBCs 7600, ESR 29, film microcytic hypochromic anaemia.

CASE G.   Hb 12.6 g, PCV 40, MCHC 32, WBCs 5600, differential count normal, ESR 46.

CASE H.   Hb 14.7 g, PCV 45, WBCs 13 600 — 80% neutrophils, ESR 30.

CASE I.   Hb 14 g, WBCs 16 300 — 90% neutrophils, ESR 24.

CASE J.   Full blood-count normal, ESR 36.

CASE K   Hb 9.6 g, hypochromic anaemia, WBCs 3800, ESR 36.

CASE L.   Hb 12.2 g, ESR 42, white cells and platelets normal.

CASE M.   Hb 7.6 g, MCH 30, MCHC 36, MCV 80, WBCs 7000, reduced platelets.

Other features will be found on pages:

CASE N.   Hb 14.6 g, WBCs 8000, platelets and film normal.

CASE O.   Hb 12.7 g, WBCs 6000, platelets normal.

CASE P.   Hb 10.7 g, MCHC 29, WBCs 8000, normal differential count, ESR 45.

CASE Q.   Hb 12.9 g, ESR 12, white cells 6000.

CASE R.   Hb 14 g, WBCs 5000, ESR 12.

CASE S.   Slight normocytic normochromic anaemia.

CASE T.   Hb 13.8 g, WBCs 12 000 − 75% neutrophils, bleeding time and clotting time normal, Hess' test positive.

CASE U.   Hb 14.2 g, WBCs 7000, normal differential count.

CASE V.   Hb 11.6 g, WBCs 7900, increased eosinophils.

CASE W.   Hb 9.6 g, WBCs 6000, normal differential count.

CASE X.   Hb 12.9 g, ESR 36, WBCs 7600, normal differential count.

CASE Y.   Hb 8.6 g, normochromic normocytic anaemia, platelets normal, WBCs 7000 normal differential count, ESR 110 mm in 1 hour.

CASE Z.   Hb 13 g, WBCs 3800, ESR 20, film normal, platelets normal.

CASE A.   Electrolytes and urea normal, liver function test normal.

CASE B.   Electrolytes and urea normal, protein-bound iodine 13.1 μg/100 ml.

CASE C.   Electrolytes, urea and liver function test normal, prothrombin ratio 5.2:1.

CASE D.   Electrolytes normal, calcium 2.8 mmol/litre, phosphorus 1.1 mmol/litre, urea normal, alkaline phosphatase 14.1 KA units, other liver-function tests normal.

CASE E.   Electrolytes normal, liver function test — bilirubin 45 mmol/litre, alkaline phosphatase 18.5 KA units, turbidity test normal, albumin 32, globulin 27 g/litre, amylase 220 Somogyi units.

CASE F.   Electrolytes, urea and liver function test normal.

CASE G.   Electrolytes and urea normal, albumin 32, globulin 41 g/litre.

CASE H.   Electrolytes and urea normal.

CASE I.   Urea and electrolytes normal.

CASE J.   Electrolytes normal, calcium 2.9 mmol/litre, phosphate 1.3 mmol/litre, alkaline phosphatase 28 KA units, parathormone level within normal limits.

CASE K.   Electrolytes normal.

CASE L.   Liver function test — alkaline phosphatase 16 KA units, transaminase normal. Calcium 2.3 mmol/litre, phosphate 1.0 mmol/litre, 5 HIAA 20 units %.

CASE M.   Electrolytes — sodium 123, potassium 6.5, chloride 110, bicarbonate 12, urea 82 mmol/litre, calcium 2.0 mmol/litre, phosphate 1.7 mmol/litre, acid phosphatase 2.6 units.

CASE N.   Electrolytes and urea normal, CSF protein 0.98 g/litre.

CASE O.   Electrolytes and urea normal, alkaline phosphatase normal.

CASE P.   Electrolytes and urea normal.

CASE Q.   Electrolytes normal, urea 10 mmol/litre.

CASE R.   Urea and electrolytes normal, calcium and phosphorus normal, alkaline phosphatase 17 KA units.

CASE S.   Electrolytes and urea normal.

CASE T.   Electrolytes and urea normal.

CASE U.   Electrolytes and urea normal.

CASE V.   Electrolytes and urea normal, bilirubin 40 mmol/litre, alkaline phosphatase 20 KA units.

CASE W.   Electrolytes and urea normal.

CASE X.   Electrolytes and urea normal, calcium 2.7 mmol/litre, alkaline phosphatase 17 KA units.

CASE Y.   Urea and electrolytes normal, plasma proteins 110 g/litre, globulin 82 g, EPS — marked increase in beta-globulins, alkaline phosphatase 12 KA units, calcium 2.8 mmol/litre, phosphorus 1.1 mmol/litre.

CASE Z.   Urea and electrolytes normal, bilirubin 14 mmol/litre, alkaline phosphatase 18 KA units, SGOT 360 units, albumin 31 g/litre, prothrombin time prolonged.

CASE A.   MSU — sterile, no cells. Sputum — sterile. Stool culture — no pathogens.

CASE B.   Normal.

CASE C.   Urine microscopy — RBCs ++, no growth.

CASE D.   Pleural effusion blood-stained, culture — no growth.

CASE E.   Urine — sterile. Sputum — moderate *H. influenzae*.

CASE F.   Urine — sterile.

CASE G.   Sputum — sterile. No AAFB. Urine — RBCs numerous, no WBCs or growth.

CASE H.   Normal.

CASE I.   Urine — pus cells ++, culture — *Proteus* species.

CASE J.   Sputum cytology — normal. Urine — increased WBCs, normal culture.

CASE K.   Urine — sterile.

CASE L.   Normal.

CASE M.   Normal.

Other features will be found on pages:

CASE N.   Normal.

CASE O.   Sputum cytology and bacteriology normal.

CASE P.   ZN stain of sputum showed AAFB. Cytology — no malignant cells.

CASE Q.   None done.

CASE R.   Sputum grew *Streptococcus pneumonii*. Cytology showed oat cell carcinoma.

CASE S.   None done.

CASE T.   Urine microscopy — RBCs ++, no WBCs or culture.

CASE U.   CSF heavily blood-stained.

CASE V.   Sputum culture normal.

CASE W.   Urine showed RBCs ++, WBCs +, no growth.

CASE X.   Urine and sputum — no growth.

CASE Y.   Marrow showed plasma cells +, urine normal.

CASE Z.   Sputum grew non-haemolytic streptococcus, MSU — sterile.

CASE A.   Chest X-ray — slight cardiomegaly, lung fields clear. Abdominal X-ray — normal.

CASE B.   Anterior mediastinal mass below thoracic inlet. Chest X-ray otherwise normal.

CASE C.   Normal.

CASE D.   Right pleural effusion ++. X-ray of upper right humerus showed osteolytic area and pathological fracture.

CASE E.   Chest X-ray — slight cardiomegaly, moderate emphysema. X-ray of abdomen — normal.

CASE F.   X-rays normal.

CASE G.   Chest X-ray showed old cavity right apex, no active tuberculosis, heart normal.

CASE H.   Chest X-ray showed dextrocardia.

CASE I.   Abdominal X-ray showed a 1-cm calculus over the right sacro-iliac joint.

CASE J.   Chest X-ray normal. X-ray of abdomen showed opacity at the tip of the 4th lumbar transverse process on the left side.

CASE K.   Chest X-ray normal. X-ray of abdomen showed an enlarged liver.

CASE L.   Chest X-ray showed right ventricular hypertrophy.

CASE M.   Moderate cardiomegaly and basal pulmonary oedema.

CASE N.   Skull and chest X-ray normal. Coned view showed some erosion of the petrous portion of the temporal bone on the left side.

CASE O.   Chest X-ray showed 'cannon-ball' secondary deposits in both lung fields.

CASE P.   Chest X-ray showed bilateral apical opacities, the right side showing some cavitation. X-ray of spine showed anterior wedging of T10 and 11. AP view suggests paravertebral abscess.

CASE Q.   Chest X-ray showed slight cardiomegaly, lung fields clear.

CASE R.   Chest X-ray showed small dense irregular right hilar opacity.

CASE S.   Chest X-ray showed widening of the mediastinum with increased hilar nodes.

CASE T.   Chest X-ray normal. Abdominal X-ray showed generalised small-bowel distension with a few fluid levels.

CASE U.   Chest X-ray and skull X-ray normal.

CASE V.   Chest X-ray normal. Abdominal X-ray showed an enlarged liver with some spherical calcification in the right lobe.

CASE W.   Chest X-ray normal. Abdominal X-ray showed gas shadows pushed to the right iliac fossa by a large opaque mass.

CASE X.   Chest X-ray showed bilateral hilar lymphadenopathy.

CASE Y.   Chest X-ray normal. X-ray of spine showed diffuse osteoporosis with some mottled areas in the upper lumbar spine.

CASE Z.   Chest X-ray showed bilateral emphysema, X-ray of abdomen showed slight hepatosplenomegaly.

CASE A.   Barium enema — multiple polyps in the colon and rectum, large carcinoma of descending colon.

CASE B.   None done.

CASE C.   Barium enema — diverticulosis of the sigmoid colon.

CASE D.   None done.

CASE E.   Barium meal — widening of the duodenal loop, otherwise normal.

CASE F.   Barium swallow — hold-up of barium in the post-cricoid region. Irregular stricture, probably carcinoma.

CASE G.   IVP — left kidney and calyces displaced and stretched.

CASE H.   None done.

CASE I.   IVP shows right pelvic kidney with a stone in the pelvis of the kidney. Left kidney normal.

CASE J.   IVP shows right hydronephrosis above calculus. Barium meal demonstrates a duodenal ulcer.

CASE K.   None done.

CASE L.   Liver scan — multiple filling defects.

CASE M.   Barium meal and follow-through normal.

CASE N.   None done.

CASE O.   IVP shows right hydronephrosis, ureter dilated to level of L4, no stone demonstrated. (?) Extrinsic compression. Barium enema — caecum displaced by retroperitoneal mass. Barium meal and follow-through normal.

CASE P.   Myelogram — compression of the spinal cord at T10, T11.

CASE Q.   IVP shows bilateral polycystic kidneys.

CASE R.   None done.

CASE S.   Barium meal — some hold-up of barium in the mid-mediastinum, no intrinsic lesion.

CASE T.   None done.

CASE U.   Carotid arteriography demonstrates a cerebral angioma.

CASE V.   Intravenous cholangiogram normal.

CASE W.   IVP shows a non-functioning left kidney, normal right kidney.

CASE X.   None done.

CASE Y.   None done.

CASE Z.   Barium meal shows oesophageal varices and possible gastric ulcer on the lesser curve.

CASE A.   Biopsy left supraclavicular node showed poorly differentiated adenocarcinoma.

CASE B.   None done.

CASE C.   Not done.

CASE D.   Biopsy lymph node left axilla — poorly differentiated carcinoma.

CASE E.   Node biopsy — adenocarcinoma.

CASE F.   Oesophagoscopy and biopsy of squamous cell carcinoma at the level of the post-cricoid region.

CASE G.   None done.

CASE H.   None done.

CASE I.   Not done.

CASE J.   None done.

CASE K.   Biopsy of groin demonstrated malignant melanoma on the right side.

CASE L.   None done.

CASE M.   None done.

CASE N.   Biopsy of nodule right arm shows a neurofibroma.

CASE O.   None done.

CASE P.   None done.

CASE Q.   None done.

CASE R.   Biopsy left supraclavicular lymph node shows oat cell carcinoma.

CASE S.   Biopsy of lymph nodes of neck demonstrated Hodgkin's disease.

CASE T.   None done.

CASE U.   None done.

CASE V.   Biopsy not done. Casoni test positive. Liver scan showed a large cold area in the right lobe.

CASE W.   None done.

CASE X.   Scaly node biopsy shows sarcoidosis.

CASE Y.   None done.

CASE Z.   None done.

Other features will be found on pages:

CASE A.   *Familial polyposis coli with malignant change descending colon.*
The patient has metastases in the liver, supraclavicular fossa, and left axilla. He is
also anaemic and in congestive failure due to the anaemia. The clues to this case are
in the strong family history. Notice the history of 'piles', which was bleeding and
mucus from the polyps. Note that the malignant change takes place at a very early
age.

CASE B.   *Secondary thyrotoxicosis with cardiac failure.* Note the long history
of multinodular goitre which is incidentally retrosternal in part. Secondary thyrotoxicosis in middle-aged patients tends to present with cardiac features rather than
with features of hypermetabolism. Notice the fibrillation and congestive failure.
This patient had some exophthalmos which is unusual with secondary thyrotoxicosis. She also had incidental haemorrhoids.

CASE C.   *Bleeding diverticular disease precipitated by Warfarin overdose.* This
patient was anticoagulated for a deep vein thrombosis; bruising and massive bleeding *per rectum* was precipitated by Warfarin overdose. She had coincidental
fibroids. With vitamin K_1 the anticoagulants were reversed. Operation to stop
bleeding was not necessary.

CASE D.   *Pathological fracture right humerus from carcinoma of breast.* Bones
are a common site for secondaries in carcinoma of the breast, but it is unusual for
the bony secondaries to be the first presentation of the disease. Note the family
history. This patient also had anaemia, hypercalcaemia producing headaches and
nausea. She had a malignant pleural effusion and metastases in the left axilla,
peritoneal cavity and liver. The management would be internal fixation of the right
humerus, possible local radiotherapy, and then hormone therapy.

CASE E.   *Thrombophlebitis migrans secondary to carcinoma of the pancreas.*
There is an increased risk of thrombo-embolism with any visceral carcinoma. This
patient had the classical Trousseau sign. Note the metastases in the left supraclavicular fossa. There was incidentally a history of old myocardial infarction. The
patient was hypertensive and had emphysema.

CASE F.   *Post-cricoid carcinoma secondary to Plummer–Vinson syndrome.*
Note the features of Plummer–Vinson syndrome — koilonychia, angular stomatitis,
iron deficiency anaemia. The anaemia was apparently secondary to her menorrhagia
and had produced a degree of congestive cardiac failure. The carcinoma developed
secondary to a post-cricoid web.

CASE G.   *Left renal adenocarcinoma* producing acute left varicocoele and
pyrexia of unknown origin. Left renal carcinoma is a rare cause of left varicocoele,
and may occasionally present with pyrexia of unknown origin. Note the coincidental old pulmonary tuberculosis and cirrhosis.

CASE H.   *Appendicitis developing in a patient with situs inversus.* This is a rare oddity; the feature that gives away the diagnosis is the finding of a dextrocardia, which may or may not be associated with situs inversus, but on finding a patient with dextrocardia the next thing is to find out on which side the liver is situated. Note the coincidental port-wine naevus of face.

CASE I.   *Acute pyelonephritis secondary to a right renal stone developing in a pelvic kidney*. The commonest cause of a tender mass in the right iliac fossa is an appendix mass. Dysuria and numerous pus cells in the urine can occur in appendicitis but the temperature here is suspiciously high and the presence of a calculus on plain film makes an alternative diagnosis likely.

CASE J.   *Primary hyperparathyroidism*. Note the common presentation with renal stone, the raised serum calcium and low phosphate. Note the parathormone level — any detectable parathormone in the blood in the presence of hypercalcaemia strongly suggests hyperparathyroidism (as hypercalcaemia normally suppresses parathormone secretion). Note the bone changes in the tibia; it is uncommon for bone and renal complications to occur together. There is an increased incidence of peptic ulceration in patients with hyperparathyroidism.

CASE K.   *Malignant melanoma, left inguinal hernia*. This patient had malignant lymph nodes in the right groin secondary to the malignant melanoma on the sole of the foot. The left groin lump was a left inguinal hernia.

CASE L.   *Carcinoid syndrome*. Note the bouts of episodic diarrhoea. There was no evidence of local colonic disease such as ulcerative colitis. The features that suggest carcinoid syndrome are the attacks of flushing, often precipitated by alcohol. Note the liver enlargement. Most patients with carcinoid syndrome have liver metastases. Note the clinical features of tricuspid incompetence which can occur secondary to carcinoid tumours. The diagnosis is confirmed by the elevated 5-hydroxyindoleacetic acid level.

CASE M.   *Uraemia, secondary to chronic retention due to enlarged prostate*. Note the presenting features of uraemia. The onset of overflow incontinence superimposed on a history of prostatism suggests the underlying cause. Note the uraemic pericarditis and the episode of bleeding possibly due to uraemic colitis. Note the normochromic normocytic anaemia and the electrolyte changes found in uraemia. The finding of a greatly distended painless bladder confirms the likely aetiological cause for the uraemia.

CASE N.   *Acoustic neuroma secondary to neurofibromatosis*. Acoustic tumours are not uncommon in neurofibromatosis. Note the family history and the diagnostic neurofibromas on the limbs associated with cafe-au-lait spots. The diagnosis of an acoustic neuroma was confirmed by the coned views of the petrous temporal bone and the finding of a very high CSF protein. Note too the involvement of the 7th and 5th cranial nerves on that side.

CASE O.   *Teratoma of an intra-abdominal testis.* This patient had a congenital undescended testis which has a higher incidence of malignant change. The patient developed a right hydronephrosis, either from direct involvement from the tumour or para-aortic nodes. He developed lung secondaries.

CASE P.   *Pott's paraparesis.* Most cases of complications of tuberculosis in recent years are found in immigrants. Note the associated pulmonary tuberculosis, the constitutional signs of TB, the kyphoscoliosis and tenderness over the lower thoracic spine associated with weakness of the leg and sensory level. Positive culture in this case was obtained from the sputum and confirmation of the diagnosis made from typical X-ray changes in the spine.

CASE Q.   *Cerebrovascular accident secondary to hypertension and polycystic kidney.* Note the classical story of a cerebrovascular accident, the family history of kidney trouble, the bilateral irregular loin masses of polycystic kidneys.

CASE R.   *Brain secondary deposits from carcinoma of the bronchus.* Note that secondary tumours occur more commonly in the brain than primary tumours. Note the late onset of epilepsy, the history of heavy smoking and coughing. Note that before onset of the fits the patient complained of headaches and vomiting suggestive of increased intracranial pressure. This was confirmed by finding papill-oedema. Confirmation of the primary was obtained on chest X-ray and sputum cytology.

CASE S.   *Hodgkin's disease.* Note its occurrence in a young adult. This is an atypical presentation of Hodgkin's disease which usually presents with neck glands. This patient's hilar lymphadenopathy produced oesophageal compression and dysphagia and cough. Note the enlarged spleen and pruritus, the normocytic normochromic anaemia and the positive histology from biopsy of a neck gland.

CASE T.   *Henoch–Schönlein purpura.* The abdominal symptoms are pro-duced commonly in this syndrome by submucosal haemorrhages in the intestine. The clinical features that suggest the diagnosis are the characteristic rash on the legs and the history of allergy which one occasionally obtains. Note the microscopic haematuria.

CASE U.   *Sturge–Weber syndrome.* This syndrome is the combination of a port-wine naevus on the face and an angioma on the other side of the brain. The angiomas may give rise to epilepsy or subarachnoid and intracerebral bleeding in a young adult.

CASE V.   *Hydatid disease of the liver.* To make a diagnosis of hepatic hydatid disease one depends on getting a history of exposure to the disease. Note this patient's occupation. The patient commonly complains of pain over the liver which is enlarged and may produce jaundice. Note the eosinophilia. The demonstration of a cold area on the liver scan and the positive Casoni test confirm the diagnosis.

CASE W.   *Wilms' tumour*. This tumour is the commonest cause of a solid mass in the abdomen in this age group. 80 per cent of cases occur below the age of 5. The child is frequently generally unwell and the mass is noted by the parents. Note the secondary hypertension and the finding of cells in the urine. The renal origin of the tumour is confirmed by intravenous urography.

CASE X.   *Sarcoidosis*. Note the diffuse enlargement of the parotid gland, which is distinct from a parotid tumour. Note the erythema nodosum and bilateral hilar lymphadenopathy demonstrated on chest X-ray. The diagnosis was confirmed with a scalene node biopsy.

CASE Y.   *Multiple myeloma*. Backache is not an uncommon presentation for this disease. Note the patient is generally unwell with weakness, anaemia and weight loss. At this age group one thinks first of carcinoma of bronchus or prostate as the cause, but rectal examination and chest X-ray were both normal. Note the normochromic normocytic anaemia, and the very high ESR. The diagnosis is confirmed by the abnormal globulin pattern in the blood, and the sternal marrow may be typical of the disease.

CASE Z.   *Bleeding oesophageal varices*. Note the history of alcoholism and stigmata of cirrhosis. Gastroscopy confirms the diagnosis. In 50 per cent of cases the actual bleeding is from another cause.